The
PREEMIE
PRIMER

The PREEMIE PRIMER

A Complete Guide for Parents
of Premature Babies—from Birth through
the Toddler Years and Beyond

Jennifer Gunter,
MD, FRCS(C), FACOG, DABPM

Foreword by Adam Rosenberg, MD, FAAP

Da Capo
LIFE
LONG

A Member of the Perseus Books Group

Designed by Pauline Brown
Set in 10.5 point Palatino Light by the Perseus Books Group

Library of Congress Cataloging-in-Publication Data

Gunter, Jennifer.
  The preemie primer : a complete guide for parents of premature babies—from birth through the toddler years and beyond / Jennifer Gunter ; foreword by Adam Rosenberg. —1st Da Capo Press ed.
     p. cm.
  Includes bibliographical references and index.
  ISBN 978-0-7382-1393-4 (alk. paper)
  1. Premature infants—Care. 2. Premature infants—Development. I. Title.
  RJ250.3.G86 2010
  618.92'011—dc22

                                                         2010007634

First Da Capo Press edition 2010

Published by Da Capo Press
A Member of the Perseus Books Group
www.dacapopress.com

Da Capo Press books are available at special discounts for bulk purchases in the U.S. by corporations, institutions, and other organizations. For more information, please contact the Special Markets Department at the Perseus Books Group, 2300 Chestnut Street, Suite 200, Philadelphia, PA, 19103, or call (800) 810-4145, ext. 5000, or e-mail special.markets@perseusbooks.com.

10 9 8 7 6 5 4 3 2 1

For Oliver and Victor,
who continue to prove that they
were born prematurely to give other kids a chance.
And for Aidan, who was lost but not forgotten.

Contents

Foreword

The *Preemie Primer* is a unique and comprehensive review of prematurity and its consequences. For families, the book provides an accurate, single source of up-to-date information on all the acute medical problems of prematurity and the management of these problems. There are also very important chapters about caring for your baby after she is discharged from the neonatal intensive care unit (NICU) and brought home.

In addition to the extensive medical information, Dr. Gunter covers a number of important themes. First and foremost is the principle of advocating for your baby through an understanding of your baby's condition. The doctors and nurses in the NICU are skilled experts in the care of preterm infants, but they change and rotate shift to shift, day to day, and month to month. Parents spend many hours by their infants' bedsides and become intimately familiar with their babies' cues of well-being and distress. This book takes that into account and empowers parents not to simply defer to the NICU staff, but to be a participating voice in their infants' care. This is in your baby's best interest.

A second very important theme is the importance of forging a close relationship with your child's primary nursing group. The bedside nurses are the most important personnel in the NICU. They are at the bedside 24/7 caring for your baby. They will keep you updated on a daily basis about your baby's condition and progress and will provide invaluable information to the neonatologist and other physicians caring for your baby. Most NICUs have a system in which one or more nurses take your baby on as a primary patient. This means that whenever they're scheduled to work, they will care for your baby. Next to you, they'll know your baby better than anyone, and they will help you advocate for your baby.

I would add to these themes another concept that is implicit. Always feel empowered to talk with the neonatologist. He or she is supervising the care of your baby and should ensure that you understand the medical treatment plan. When you're feeling at loose ends, ask for a conference with the care team.

Advocating for your baby does not stop with NICU discharge. *The Preemie Primer* provides useful information about services available after you bring your baby home to help attain the best possible outcome. Although they may be readily available, these services are often complicated to access.

Another unique aspect of *The Preemie Primer* is the sprinkling of personal stories about Jennifer's own sons, Oliver and Victor. These vignettes make the medical information provided more real, and the suffering, uncertainty, and sometimes powerlessness of parents in an NICU more evident. Jennifer also emphasizes the very important issue of postpartum depression, which is often under-recognized by your baby's medical team. This is a real medical condition requiring treatment and can be exacerbated by having a very sick preterm infant. It's never inappropriate to ask to see a therapist or psychiatrist with expertise in the management of postpartum depression. Some NICUs have someone available. If yours does not, ask your obstetrician or NICU social worker for a referral. You are less capable of helping your baby if you're struggling emotionally.

It is very moving for me to write a foreword for this important book for parents of preterm infants. I have practiced neonatology for nearly 30 years and took part in Oliver and Victor's care in the NICU. I've always tried to be sensitive to the needs of both families and babies, but Jennifer's insights have served to make me more sensitive and aware—for that I am thankful.

I also have the good fortune to run a clinic for graduates of our NICU and was fortunate to care for Oliver and Victor until they moved away from Denver. Seeing them and the other remarkable children grow and overcome many obstacles is the most gratifying experience in my premature practice. They prove me wrong every day.

Although there were many moments of doubt, Jennifer truly maintained a glass-is-half-full approach and never hesitated for one moment to do whatever was necessary for Oliver and Victor. I'm confident that readers will learn from the book's medical knowledge and use it to be intimately involved in the care of their infants.

Adam Rosenberg, MD, FAAP
Professor, Department of Pediatrics
Division of Neonatology
University of Colorado
Denver School of Medicine

Prologue:

Our Story

There's a well-entrenched theory that OB/GYNs have the most complicated pregnancies. In reality most of us probably do not, but doctors remember complications most vividly when they happen to people they know and love. My pregnancy was, unfortunately, a good example of that old adage. Many of my colleagues who looked after me during that time have said, "It was the worst night of my life." To be remembered this way is odd, although I know they mean well.

I had been practicing OB/GYN for eight years, 13 if you consider residency, when my husband Tony and I decided we wanted a family. Things did not go as planned naturally, so after a frank discussion we decided to try one cycle of infertility treatment; if it didn't work we would adopt.

In February 2003, after a battery of blood tests, I started daily injections to try and coax my ovaries into action. My doctor tried to sound positive, but I can read ultrasounds and knew I wasn't responding well. I gave myself one cycle, and although I tried to put it out of my mind, it was difficult as there was so much time, energy, and money tightly packed in with our hopes and dreams.

I was very surprised when my cycle failed to start. Not wanting to make my disappointment public with blood work at the hospital, I took a home pregnancy test. A few minutes later I was standing in my bathroom looking at the stick, stunned beyond belief. Years of training simply vanished while I anxiously looked for a blue line. So I did a second one, and then a third to be sure.

I *was* pregnant.

And then I started to worry. I was afraid the pregnancy I had dismissed as impossible would somehow vanish. All those fears and desires I had efficiently locked away came flooding out. And then I had my first ultrasound and I realized we did have something to worry about: I was pregnant with triplets.

On July 5, 2003, when I was 22½ weeks into the pregnancy, I woke up in the middle of the night in a pool of water and knew I had ruptured my membranes. I needed a few minutes to summon my courage, so I silently sat in our bathroom staring into the night. I felt as if I were in a way station between worlds. After a few minutes I would have no option but to stand up and move on. I could see my old life, one of constancy and control, slip away into the darkness and a new existence, more painful and uncertain, emerging. I took a deep breath and walked through the door.

"We need to go the hospital right away," I said from the middle of the bedroom. My husband sat bolt upright. He could sense my harnessed panic. I knew he wanted to believe I was overreacting, that it was probably nothing, but deep down he understood.

There are no words to describe the sadness in our hearts as we drove to the hospital in the quiet of night. Just breathing seemed to be an effort, so we silently sat beside each other in the car, enveloped in a cloak of darkness and sorrow.

I wanted to believe I had somehow been mistaken, that in a few minutes we would all laugh about the OB/GYN who couldn't tell if she had ruptured her own membranes. But after the testing was complete, the doctor on call came into the room and sat on the edge of my bed. I couldn't look at Tony as we listened to the grim statistics. I had known all along what this meant, how bad it really was, but I couldn't bring myself to be the one to tell my husband. I didn't cry until I saw the look on his face.

And so I lay in a hospital bed waiting for the inevitable: to lose three boys, a whole family, at once. I imagine this is what it feels like when you're waiting for your execution but have not committed the crime. You cannot believe it's happening, but you still hold hope for a pardon that, in reality, almost never comes. We ordered pizza, friends visited, and as long as no one made eye contact, we could pretend the elephant was not in the room. All the while I couldn't forget that a storm was brewing inside of me.

And then the storm broke.

I woke up to go to the bathroom and as soon as I closed the door I knew. I was terrified to reach down and feel what my body was telling me, but I did anyway. My first son was delivering. I was shaking so hard it felt as if the earth must be shaking too. And then instinct took over and I screamed and screamed. I was still screaming inside, even after I stopped making any noise.

It was one of those moments in life when everything seems to happen in slow motion. It was probably only seconds, but it seemed like hours, and the nurse was there, catching my son with one arm and guiding me back to bed with the other. The memories of those few moments, from the act of closing the bathroom door to the delivery, are burned in my memory. I can close my eyes and see it today just as it was years ago. I can feel the cool linoleum on my feet, hear the bathroom door shut, and touch his frail body. If I don't distract myself the loop can play over and over again, like a bad movie clip.

And then the worst words that I have ever heard, "Do you want to hold your son? He is dying." How *do* you answer that question? I was too scared to make it real, to understand what I had just lost. Tony was braver and gently held Aidan. Eventually he lay in my arms, swaddled in a blanket, with a tiny, perfect face that would make you cry to look at it.

It was all too much to process. So I lay there quietly waiting for my other two boys to deliver, for this tragedy to come to fruition. And then I realized nothing was happening—it was as if my uterus had simply run out of gas. Somehow, I was still pregnant with two.

This is one of those times in medicine when there is no explanation. Usually once labor starts, all of the babies with a multiple pregnancy deliver in fairly rapid succession; however, in some cases, only one delivers and the pregnancy continues. Twenty percent of the time the remaining babies will get a week or even more inside their mothers. The process is called a **delayed-interval delivery.** Most OB/GYNs might see one or two babies survive an interval delivery in their career. I had seen a successful outcome *once*. And so I lay in bed thinking, "If she can do it, so can I."

I became fixed on getting to 26 weeks, a watershed moment in prematurity when survival improves exponentially. Over and over I told myself the three of us would see 26 weeks together. I chanted 26 weeks and meditated on it, trying to let that number sink into every cell.

To improve the odds, I had a stitch placed in my cervix and took antibiotics as well as numerous medications to try to stop my contractions. On strict bed rest, I spent my days and nights confined to my hospital bed. What I remember most from that time were the early mornings when the first rays of sunlight start to dilute the blackness ever so slightly. The new day is not here yet, but you know it's coming. I would wake at 4 AM for my early morning medication and wait for that time between night and day. As the darkness started to lift I would whisper to myself, "One day closer." It became a ritual. I always said it out loud as an affirmation. Hours became days, and that's how it went for three and a half weeks.

One day shy of that coveted 26 weeks, I developed an infection and delivery was necessary. By the time my Cesarean section was arranged, the day had turned and I was 26 weeks. Some doctors, less vested in the situation, would probably think it was simply chance. But really, what were the odds that I would deliver *exactly* at 26 weeks? Sometimes I chide myself, jokingly of course, that I should have picked 27 or 28 weeks!

Our boys, Oliver and Victor, weighed 783 grams (1 lb, 11½ oz) and 833 grams (1 lb, 13 oz), respectively, and when the doctor came to tell us how they were doing I was expecting to hear, "They're small, but look great." In my mind I had somehow convinced myself that getting to 26 weeks was all that was needed, when really it was just the beginning. The doctor explained they were much sicker than expected. I asked him if they were going to make it. His answer felt like a bucket of cold water, "A fifty-fifty chance, *maybe*." But I could tell from his look and tone that he was being generous. And I had thought the worst was over. I could not even bear to think what I would do if we lost another one.

The first few days in the neonatal intensive care unit (NICU) were strange. Being an OB/GYN seemed like a lifetime ago. Even though I had visited this place many times before checking on babies I had delivered, now that my own boys were patients, I felt like an outsider with my nose pressed up against the glass. In addition, I was sick with a serious infection, incredibly sore from the surgery, and weak from almost four weeks of bed rest, never mind the storm of hormones and emotions. In a fog of pain, sorrow, and hopelessness, I traipsed back and forth from my room to the NICU, trying not to look at the overjoyed new parents with *their* healthy babies. I felt like the only girl at the prom without a date, watching from the shadows of the gym.

Even though I was very ill with the infection, secretly I was glad, because it allowed me to stay in the hospital longer. It was a crazy thought, because these kinds of infections are one of the main reasons women die after giving birth. But that's how desperate I was to be with my babies; the thought of going home paled in comparison.

Eight days after the boys were born I was physically well enough to leave the hospital. Most new mothers get a triumphant wheelchair ride. They are like beauty pageant winners, clutching their babies instead of roses, their faces beaming with excitement while they glide through the hallways as if they were taking their first turn on the stage before an adoring crowd. But no one looks at the mother without a baby. We are the invisible.

I didn't start to unravel until I got in the car. The sound of the door closing was like a punctuation mark for all that pent-up emotion, and I began to sob. I have never felt so utterly devastated. I was crying for our son who died, for our boys who might not live, and for all the dreams that had vanished.

The doctor and nurses encouraged me to take a few days off from the intensive care unit and rest at home, but the very next day I insisted Tony take me to the hospital on his way to work, as I was still too sore to drive. Exhausted by the effort of getting dressed and walking from the car, I sat in the intensive care unit simply overwhelmed with fatigue and the gravity of the situation.

I somehow managed to summon enough strength to stumble down the hallway to labor and delivery. I found an open on-call room and lay down on an empty bed hoping to rest and cry some more. It was a very surreal moment: an OB/GYN on maternity leave sleeping in an obstetrical call room. And that was when it hit me—only a doctor would know where to find a vacant room. I had home court advantage and I needed to use it. I knew how to get things done in a hospital.

As I got physically stronger, I started to do more. Most new mothers spend their first few weeks bonding: holding their newborns, touching them, drinking them in. So I did what I could, substituting medical care such as taking their temperature and helping with their daily weigh-ins for feeding and cuddling. Sometimes I would just sit with them, because that was the only thing I could offer. When I was not physically at their bedside, I devoured textbooks and research papers on prematurity.

After a week I was allowed to hold them. I was terrified. They were so tiny, and there was so much equipment. Surely I would break them or at least disconnect all the tubes. But then I cradled them naked against my skin, and as my body provided warmth and my breathing and heart-beat more natural rhythms, their breathing became easier, their heart rates stabilized, and they needed less oxygen. It was wonderful, for me and for them, medically and emotionally. That was the moment I knew we could make a difference, that *we* were the key to their success.

For every two steps forward there was almost always a step or more backward. It's a dance that repeats itself over and over. It's hard to predict the course of events in the NICU: Premature babies write their own rules. Just when I thought things were starting to stabilize, Oliver was diagnosed with a serious heart defect and had his first of two surgeries when he was only 1,400 grams (3 lbs, 1 oz). When it seemed we were back on course again, Victor had a series of setbacks.

Eleven weeks after they were born, they both came home, but with oxygen, monitors, and numerous medications. They needed intensive follow-up and endless home interventions along with all the regular baby care that goes along with two newborns. I was fortunate enough to have an extended maternity leave, but after six months the harsh reality set in. We had deluded ourselves into thinking this around-the-clock care would magically disappear within a few months, but there was no returning to our previous life. I wanted to stay at home longer, but we couldn't afford to be without my salary anymore, so my husband quit his job. It was very hard for him, because, as with many men, his identity is intimately related to his work. He *loves* architecture.

Tony was determined to be the biggest kid in the house, and the three of them did things I never dreamed of doing. I would come home only to find they had been all over town with oxygen tanks in tow and would *freak out!* You went to the mall? (Did you take hand sanitizer?) You went to the park? (Did you take hats and sunscreen?) I taught him to be more cautious, and he taught me to let go. Without him, I'm not sure if I would have had enough courage to let them go out into the world.

Tony found new ways to express his creativity by building equipment. He has an intuitive understanding of form and function; I would talk about a new therapy, and he would quickly rig up the perfect piece of equipment in MacGyver-like fashion. He built the most amazing therapy table, adapted high chairs, and jury-rigged strollers—our physical therapist marveled at his creations.

Since the boys' discharge there have been hundreds of appointments with doctors, nurses, and therapists, in addition to emergency room visits, hospitalizations, surgeries, and even admissions to the pediatric intensive care unit. There have been other battles as well, with medical professionals, insurance companies, hospitals, and special programs. The system can be adversarial and impossible to navigate, even for an insider! The stakes are high because every missed therapy or treatment opportunity can affect your baby. At times I felt like Alice in Wonderland in court with the King and Queen of Hearts. The rules seem made up and it's all so nonsensical that you want to laugh, cry, and scream at the same time.

The standard line from doctors is that premature babies catch up with their peers by the age of two. So, we automatically assumed that all the hardships they have endured in their short lives would be magically erased when they blew out those birthday candles. The truth is that it takes a Herculean effort to help a premature baby catch up, and sadly, some never do. Doctors need to be more careful with their choice of words, because it's very easy to hear what you want and harder to face more disappointments.

There is also the all too real specter of disability. Both boys have physical challenges, and Oliver has suffered with a combination of lung damage and heart problems, enduring multiple readmissions to the hospital. However, with time and a lot of effort, things are improving. And that's the best mantra for any parent with a premature baby: time and effort.

Along the way, someone told me that the best thing you can do for your child who has limitations is to give him or her a sense of self, and our boys have that in spades. We focus on what they can do, we work on the challenges, and as they get older it's harder to see what separates them from their peers born after the full 40 weeks. Yes, prematurity adds more complexities, but parents with full-term babies also struggle. We're not so different after all. Parenting is challenging no matter how you look at it.

Years ago in my 10th-grade French class we had to give an oral report on how to do something. For most of us this involved hours of translation to produce a page or so of work. I stood in front of the class and recited, in French of course, *How to Bake Chocolate Chip Cookies*. I thought I was so smart bringing the cookies to share with the class. Then one of the quieter boys from the back stood up and informed us his essay was titled *How to Walk*. He spoke one sentence, "Put one foot in front of the other and repeat." We were all stunned, the teacher especially. The class roared. Brilliant!

Brilliant indeed.

It's funny how, years later, these childhood moments can be as vivid as the day we first lived them. When I experience this memory I feel as if I'm really there, sitting in on the class like Scrooge visiting his Christmas past. This memory has become very dear to me, even inspirational. Because that is exactly what you do in a time of crisis. You put one foot in front of the other and repeat.

PART ONE

The Beginning

I

~~~~~~~~~~

Prematurity 101

Five hundred thousand babies are born prematurely every year in the United States (approximately 12.5 percent of all births), and worldwide the numbers are in the *millions*. It is the leading cause of death and disability for newborns. However, you don't have to sit by just hoping for the best. You *can* have a positive influence on your baby's health. Countless medical studies show that parents are a key factor in improving a premature baby's chances. And that is the foundation for this book—the idea that *you* are the most integral part of your baby's health care team.

> When my boys were born I felt like Pigpen from Peanuts, except I was surrounded by a cloud of bad news instead of a cloud of dirt. I spent a lot of time in those early days wishing things were different. However, visions of the life that was not to be only left me more depressed. I needed to occupy myself, so I went to my office (one floor above the NICU) and started to research prematurity. I found that salvation from my sadness and turmoil lay in the science. There were medical therapies and interventions to give a baby the best chance. I wasn't as helpless or ineffectual as I thought.
>
> I tried to reframe my thoughts. When I was told, "There is a 50 percent chance your boys will live," I heard, "There is a 50 percent chance your boys will live *and* it takes something to be in the right 50 percent, so let's get started!" I began to think about the information actively, not passively. If a good (or at least better) outcome was possible, I figured that it might as well be my boys who got it, and so my motto became *focus forward*, no matter how bad the news. It helped me feel as if I were heading toward something, instead of running away.

Can I Really Learn This?

Prematurity is complex, even for doctors. Some medical professionals worry that the information is too difficult or stressful for parents. However, understanding medicine is a bit like learning to bake. If you understand the basics and have the right recipe, ingredients, and tools, you can bake almost anything. The more you bake, the more complex the recipes you can tackle. This book will provide you with the right medical building blocks, and with it you will be able to expand your knowledge, learning what you need to know to help your baby.

What about the idea that the information is just too frightening? Medical studies indicate that parents of premature babies want empowering information. Being uninformed leaves parents disconnected and helpless. Think back to any other problem in your life. Have you ever said, "I wish I had been less prepared?" Probably not.

There *will* be times when the information and statistics are overwhelming. Go at a pace that works for you. It's also important to keep in mind that this book discusses many medical challenges, but that does not mean they will all happen to your baby. Try to limit your worry to what you know for sure. You have enough on your plate.

Learning about your baby's medical needs and getting involved is empowering and will make you feel more connected. But most important, you will actually improve your baby's chances of living her best life, and *that* is what parenting is all about.

Getting Started

There are three core essentials for helping your baby:

- **Knowledge.** When you are informed, you feel empowered, communicate more effectively with the medical team, have a better chance of improving the variables under your control, and acquire an understanding of things that cannot be changed.

- **Advocacy.** You are your baby's team leader. Being proactive and involved improves outcomes and is also empowering.
- **Just being there.** Being around and interacting with your baby is healing for both of you. In addition, premature babies often do not appear ill until they are very sick, so parents who learn their baby's nuances may be able to spot minor changes earlier.

What Does Prematurity Mean?

The due date for a pregnancy is 40 weeks, but that is an approximate date, as a **full-term** delivery can happen anytime between 37 and 42 weeks. Babies born before 37 weeks are premature. Growing and developing in the outside world as opposed to the protective environment of the uterus has effects on almost every organ system and also affects the ability of a baby to gain weight and grow.

When doctors speak about the ramifications of prematurity, they will specifically talk about three things:

- **The chance of surviving.**
- **The possibility of major complications,** meaning significant lung damage, serious bowel problems, nervous system issues, or problems with vision. These complications have the biggest impact on survival and disability.
- **The risk of disability.** Disability means impairment of body function or structure. It is a broad term that encompasses any type of limitation, from attention deficit disorder to cerebral palsy.

The information you receive from the medical team is a *best guess* based on studies that look at thousands of premature babies. It's important to remember that these statistics reflect the odds something *could* happen, not the certainty that it *will.* After your baby is born, the medical team will be able to fill in more of the blanks, but unfortunately what you *want* to know will only come with time.

The most significant factor in predicting the outcome for your baby is gestational age, meaning how far along in the pregnancy you are at delivery. Gestational age is calculated from the first date of the last menstrual period (LMP) or by an ultrasound between 8 and 13 weeks. It is more precise to use weeks and days, such as 27 weeks and 4 days (also written as 27⁴), instead of months, as the number of days per month varies, and sometimes a few days makes a big difference. Premature babies are divided by gestational age into four groups:

1. **Late preterm, 34–36⁶ weeks.** More than 70 percent of premature babies are in this group. Major complications are rare. The most common issues are transient breathing problems, the buildup of a toxin in the blood called **bilirubin** (jaundice), and insufficient weight gain. Some late preterm babies will go to a regular nursery with full-term babies, but others will need observation or treatment in an intensive care setting.

2. **Moderately preterm, 32–33⁶ weeks.** These babies need close monitoring of oxygen levels, heart rate, body temperature, and blood pressure. Many will need oxygen for breathing, and most will be fed with a tube. Major complications can happen, but they are uncommon. The biggest issues to monitor are lung problems, infection, weight gain, feeding, jaundice, and the development of the nervous system.

3. **Very preterm, 28–31⁶ weeks.** Any baby born before 32 weeks will need intensive care. Many will need oxygen or even special equipment to breathe. These babies are at risk for problems involving the lungs, nervous system, gastrointestinal tract, and vision in addition to infection, feeding issues, insufficient weight gain, and jaundice.

4. **Extremely preterm, less than 28 weeks.** These babies require special care for almost every bodily function we take for granted. Each additional week of prematurity has a significant impact on survival and the risk of disability. (See Table 1.) For babies between 22 and 25⁶, more individualized information is available by con-

TABLE 1: Outcomes for Extremely Preterm Babies Based on Gestational Age

Gestational age	Survival	Severe or moderate disability among survivors	Minor disability among survivors
Full term	>99%	1%	8%
34–36[6] weeks	>99%	4%	15%
32–33[6] weeks	>98%	8%	15%
28–31[6] weeks	95%	12%	25%
27–27[6] weeks	90%	25%	25%
26–26[6] weeks	85%	25%	25%
25–25[6] weeks	60–75%	30%	30%
24–24[6] weeks	26–60%	>30%	>30%
23–23[6]	8–33%	>30%	>30%
22–22[6]	< 20%	Insufficient medical studies to provide specific numbers, as very few of these babies survive.	

sidering four variables: birth weight (bigger is better), gender (girls do better), single or multiple pregnancy (one baby has the best chance), and whether the mom received steroids (special medication to help a baby's lungs mature). While these variables actually affect outcome for all premature babies, they have the greatest impact at this extreme of prematurity. Having all four of these advantages—a well-grown girl from a single pregnancy whose mother received steroids—is the equivalent of adding an extra week. The National Institutes of Health (NIH) provides a tool for doctors to more accurately calculate the odds of survival and serious disability for babies between 22 and 25[6] weeks. (Link available at www.preemieprimer.com.)

I understand how heart wrenching it is to be at the very worst end of the statistics. When my membranes ruptured at 22^5 weeks, my boys faced a 3 percent chance of survival without a serious disability. I knew there were stories of miracle babies, but that was not the reality for 97 percent of families in our situation. We decided not to pursue care. I lost a piece of my soul when we let Aidan go, but for us it was the right decision. Another family in the same situation might feel differently. It's agonizing and unfair, but nothing about prematurity is fair. You will cry and you will feel as if your heart is breaking, because it is, regardless of what you decide.

Parenting is caring and loving, and in these most trying of times we show how much we care and the depth of our love the best way that we can. All you can ask of yourself is to promise to do your best. For every one of us that will mean something different, but sometimes that is all you have, and that's okay.

Understanding Disability

To hear your baby's chance of living or risk of disability distilled to a grim statistic is heartbreaking. However, these discussions are needed, no matter how difficult, because you need to know what might lie ahead. What makes it even harder is the fact that the full ramifications of a premature delivery are not known for many years, and the unknown is scary.

Before you read further, it's important to remember that your baby is not defined by a diagnosis. A diagnosis is just a point on a map. It is information to help you get where you are going, which is the best possible life for your child.

Disability generally applies to a problem with the nervous system, vision, or hearing. It's divided into the following three groups:

- **Severe disability,** meaning physical conditions that preclude the ability to live independently, serious intellectual limitations, blindness, or profound deafness.

- **Moderate disability,** meaning independent living is possible with modifications or aids, the IQ is significantly lower than expected, vision is impaired without blindness, or there is hearing loss that can be corrected with aids.
- **Mild disability,** which applies to limitations that have a minor impact on everyday living. Many are not visible to the untrained eye, but may still be challenging. Examples include problems co-ordinating finger movements (fine motor skills), behavior issues, or learning difficulties.

For many children prematurity will leave no residual effects, and for others it will, with some more severely affected than others. However, babies also have an amazing capacity for adaptation. With time, therapies, and the right environment, progress is often possible. This catch-up can continue through childhood and even into adolescence, but it takes constant vigilance with medical care, therapies, and exercises to get the best outcome.

Having a disability means some aspects of life will be harder, but if you believe that your child cannot succeed, what chance will she have? You can take a negative approach or you can face the challenges head-on and figure out how to get the best out of life. Children are very perceptive, even as babies, and they will learn from your example.

When a Baby Is Just Too Premature

Some parents with premature babies face the most agonizing of decisions. The chance of survival or severe disability may be so grim due to early gestational age, low birth weight, infection, or any number of other horrible circumstances, that the medical team may discuss providing only comfort measures at birth, knowing that a baby this sick will succumb very quickly.

Your doctors will try their best to give you the most accurate information, but they cannot tell you what to do. They are not the ones who have to say good-bye, sit beside a crib in the intensive care unit for months, or take home a baby who is profoundly impaired.

There is no easy answer and no right or wrong. Some parents feel that they must proceed with all care regardless of the odds, while others believe the very real potential of months of intensive care followed by a life of severe, profound disability is not in their child's best interest.

~~~~~~~~~~~~~~~~

Causes of Prematurity
and Interventions

There are many medical conditions that contribute to prematurity. Premature delivery may be recommended, either for your health or the health of your baby (also called an **indicated delivery**), or it may happen spontaneously. With a spontaneous delivery, sometimes the cause is clear, but more often than not there is a complex interplay of several medical conditions, and the exact cause of the premature delivery is unknown.

Preterm Labor

Preterm labor is diagnosed when contractions cause your cervix to thin and dilate before 37 weeks. This is the most common reason for a premature delivery. Ruptured membranes or an infection may trigger preterm labor, or there may be no obvious cause.

The warning signs of preterm labor include cramps, contractions, pelvic pressure, or a change in vaginal discharge. Some women have episodic back pain. While these symptoms are not a reliable way to diagnose preterm labor (they are very common in pregnancies that deliver at term), they should be evaluated to see if they are associated with a change in cervical length, texture, and dilation.

The most reliable way to exclude preterm labor is a vaginal swab called a **fetal fibronectin test.** Fetal fibronectin is a protein that works like glue to keep the membranes attached to the inside of your uterus. If this glue becomes damaged by contractions, it leaks into the vagina. A negative test means the chance of delivering prematurely within the next seven days is less than 1 percent. A fetal fibronectin test will likely not be performed if your cervix is more than 3 cm in length, as it adds no information with a long cervix. If you test positive, it may mean that your risk of delivering in the next seven days is increased. Observation in the hospital may be recommended for closer monitoring and possible interventions, such as:

- **Testing and treatment for group B streptococcus** or group B strep (GBS), a bacteria present in the vaginal secretions of up to 25 percent of healthy women. All pregnant women are routinely checked at 35 to 37 weeks of pregnancy. If you have preterm labor prior to this time period, you will be tested, because exposure to GBS during delivery can produce life-threatening infections for your baby. Intravenous antibiotics in labor will reduce your baby's risk of infection.
- **Magnesium sulfate,** a medication given to mom to reduce her premature baby's risk of cerebral palsy. *Magnesium sulfate* is only recommended for preterm labor at less than 32–34 weeks.
- **Administering tocolytics,** which are medications to stop labor. The most effective medications are *indomethacin* and *nifedipine*. *Magnesium sulfate* may sometimes work as a tocolytic. If *magnesium sulfate* is given to prevent cerebral palsy but labor does not stop, *indomethacin* is the safest tocolytic to combine with *magnesium sulfate.* The best a tocolytic can do is stop labor for about 48 hours, long enough for the mother to receive corticosteroids or to be transferred to another medical center.
- **Injections of corticosteroids,** hormones you receive (if you are less than 34 weeks) to reduce the risk of lung, nervous system, and bowel complications. It takes 48 hours after the first dose for the

maximum benefit to be effected. Even if delivery seems imminent, it is still worth giving steroids, as some medication reaches the baby within an hour.

Preterm Premature Rupture of Membranes

In an uneventful pregnancy, the membranes protecting the baby in the womb will rupture at 37 to 42 weeks, either right before or during labor. **Preterm premature rupture of membranes,** or **PPROM,** is diagnosed when the membranes rupture before 37 weeks. The most common causes are premature labor and infection, both of which weaken the membranes. Smoking and certain vitamin deficiencies also affect membrane strength and the risk of PPROM.

PPROM is concerning for several reasons:

- **The risk of delivery is high.** Chemicals that trigger labor are released when the membranes rupture. Most babies deliver within the first week after PPROM.
- **Infection (also called chorioamnionitis) may occur,** as the physical barrier to bacteria is gone.
- **Oxygen delivery may be affected.** When the amniotic fluid is very low, the umbilical cord can become compressed, decreasing the flow of oxygen to your baby.
- **Lung complications can arise** because adequate amniotic fluid is essential for lung development. PPROM before 28 weeks is of particular concern for the lungs.
- **Separation of the placenta from the wall of the uterus, or abruption, may occur.** This is caused by the rapid decompression of the uterus as the amniotic fluid leaks out.

The diagnosis of PPROM can be difficult. You may not know exactly what is leaking: amniotic fluid, urine, or vaginal discharge. Low fluid detected on ultrasound may suggest PPROM, but the diagnosis is confirmed with a pelvic exam: your doctor will insert a speculum (the instrument used for a Pap smear) and look for fluid coming out of the cervix. Testing will confirm whether it is amniotic fluid.

Once you're diagnosed with PPROM, you will be admitted to the hospital and placed on bed rest, which may help your fluid re-accumulate. Other treatments may include:

- **Close monitoring** to assess your baby's health, the re-accumulation of amniotic fluid, and any signs of labor or infection.
- **Antibiotics** for seven days, which decreases the risk of infection and of delivering in the next three weeks.
- **Group B strep (GBS) testing and treatment.** The antibiotics that you receive in the first seven days will also treat group B strep. If you do not deliver within the first week and are group B strep positive, appropriate antibiotics must be re-started when you do go into labor.
- **Corticosteroids,** recommended if you experience PPROM before 32 to 34 weeks, as the risk of delivery within the next seven days is high.
- *Magnesium sulfate* to reduce the risk of cerebral palsy.
- **Tocolytics,** which may be indicated if labor starts, to try to delay delivery long enough to administer steroids. Tocolytics should not be given if you have an infection.
- **Delivery.** Because the risk of infection is so great with PPROM, premature delivery is usually recommend at 34 weeks. If you develop an infection, regardless of gestational age, you must be delivered.

Infection

Infection of the membranes, placenta, and amniotic fluid is called chorioamnionitis. The source is almost always bacteria from the vagina, which seep up behind the membranes into the uterus, spreading to the placenta and then to both mom and baby. Chorioamnionitis can cause

After I completed my seven days of antibiotics, my obstetrician discussed discontinuing them. I knew the data—one week of antibiotics. Long enough to hopefully get three extra weeks of pregnancy but short enough to prevent antibiotics resistance, an increasing problem in which antibiotics become less and less effective against bacteria.

In spite of my expert knowledge, I wanted to take the antibiotics for longer. Lying in my hospital bed, left to my own thoughts, I had worked out a completely illogical scenario with antibiotics as my savior. I was terrified about changing any part of the routine. Surely my case was different. Shouldn't we bend the rules for me?

My doctor listened patiently. To his credit, he worked the conversation around so it was my idea to stop the antibiotics. That night, I lay awake staring into the darkness convinced every twinge was a contraction, a portent of the infection brewing inside. The night seemed to crawl along until dawn, but when the sun came up, I was still pregnant.

In the end, the recommended seven-day regimen helped give me the three weeks I needed. The risks of a longer course of antibiotics became clear when I developed a resistant infection after my C-section. There were still a couple of effective antibiotics, but that might not have been the case had I continued the antibiotics for longer.

Because there is often little to offer, it's easy to think more is better. This makes stopping a treatment, especially when it's the last option, very difficult.

premature labor and PPROM, but may also have very few symptoms. Risk factors include a short cervix, a bacterial imbalance in the vagina, and nutritional issues, although it's unusual to find a specific cause.

Chorioamnionitis occurs in approximately 30 percent of premature deliveries, so it should always be suspected. Specific signs include fever, a tender belly, a rapid heart rate for you and/or your baby, and foul-smelling or thick, yellowish vaginal discharge. Blood tests may help, but the definitive test for chorioamnionitis is an *amniocentesis*, removing a small amount of amniotic fluid with a needle and testing it for evidence of infection.

The treatment of chorioamnionitis includes:

- **Corticosteroids.**
- **Antibiotics.** They can help reduce complications, but this type of infection is not possible to treat completely, for either you or your baby, while you are pregnant.
- **Delivery** regardless of gestational age, and even if you have no symptoms. Despite antibiotics, the bacteria will spread from your uterus to you and your baby, making you both very sick. If the infection reaches your baby's bloodstream, her risk of serious lung problems, cerebral palsy, and other complications increases significantly.

Cervical Insufficiency

A normal cervix is 3.5 to 5 cm long when measured by transvaginal ultrasound (the most accurate method of measuring it). Cervical insufficiency is diagnosed when your cervix is less than 2.5 cm in length on ultrasound in the second trimester *without* contractions or cramping. If your cervix is less than 2.5 cm, the risk of a premature delivery is 18 percent and if your cervix is less than 1.5 cm in length, the risk increases to 33 percent.

Cervical insufficiency is not caused by normal activities such as exercise, heavy lifting, or intercourse. For most women, the cervix is simply weak, although injury from surgery or a previous delivery can increase your risk. Cervical insufficiency is painless, so there are no warning signs. It's often diagnosed during a routine pelvic exam or ultrasound.

If your doctor suspects cervical insufficiency, you'll be admitted to the hospital, as delivery can happen very quickly. Specific therapies depend on age and may include:

- **Bed rest** to take weight off your cervix.
- **Abstaining from intercourse,** as sex can introduce infection.
- **Monitoring for signs of labor and infection.**

- **Ultrasound measurements of your cervix.**
- *Magnesium sulfate* to protect against cerebral palsy.
- **Progesterone,** which is a hormone made by the placenta. A progesterone vaginal suppository every night may reduce your risk of delivering prematurely if your cervix is less than 1.5 cm.
- **A stitch to strengthen the cervix,** also called a **cerclage.** Because there is risk of rupturing the membranes or introducing infection, cerclage is only considered if the cervix is 1.5 cm or less, meaning the risk of delivery is high, and delivery would be catastrophic (typically between 22 and 24 weeks). Cerclage is also performed between 13 and 16 weeks to prevent preterm delivery for women with a history of cervical insufficiency. The risks with an early cerclage are much lower.

Intrauterine Growth Restriction

Intrauterine growth restriction (IUGR) is diagnosed when your baby is among the smallest 10 percent. (This is also called the 10th percentile; the 50th percentile is average.) The most common cause is reduced oxygen delivery to the baby due to a placenta that has been damaged by high blood pressure, other medical conditions, or smoking. Other causes of IUGR include infection and genetic conditions. IUGR increases your baby's risk of complications after delivery and in some cases may increase your risk of stillbirth. The more growth restricted your baby, the greater these risks.

Your doctor will suspect IUGR if your belly is measuring smaller than expected, but an ultrasound is required for the diagnosis. An ultrasound can also evaluate blood flow to and from your baby as well as the volume of amniotic fluid, another sign of placental health.

Once the diagnosis of IUGR is confirmed, it's important to identify a cause. The ultrasound will provide a lot of information about the health of your placenta and the flow of blood to your baby. Blood tests will tell if you have been exposed to viruses that can cause IUGR. An amniocentesis may also be recommended to test for viruses and genetic conditions.

Close monitoring of your baby's health is essential. This will include:

- **A non-stress test (NST),** which is a recording of your baby's heartbeat and your uterine contractions. You will click a button every time you feel your baby move. A heart rate between 120 and 160 beats per minute that increases with movement is reassuring.
- **A biophysical profile (BPP),** which is a dynamic assessment of your baby's health that combines ultrasound and an NST. A BPP looks at a set of specific movements and at the amniotic fluid. It is scored on a scale of 2 to 10; scores of 8 and higher are reassuring.
- **Ultrasounds** every two to four weeks to monitor your baby's growth.

There are no therapies to reverse IUGR, with the exception of quitting smoking. Nutrition should be optimized (a dietician may be helpful) and bed rest may improve weight gain. If growth is too slow or if the testing of your baby's health is not reassuring, then delivery will be recommended.

If you are less than 32–34 weeks and a premature delivery is indicated for IUGR (or for any other condition), steroids and *magnesium sulfate* may be administered before delivery to improve your baby's outcome.

Pre-eclampsia

Pre-eclampsia is a medical condition in which high blood pressure, swelling, and protein in the urine develop *after* 20 weeks. It affects 5 percent of pregnancies and is the result of abnormal blood vessels in the placenta. For some women it is a mild condition, but for others it can lead to stroke, seizures, damage to the internal organs, excessive bleeding, and even death. The damaged placenta can also lead to low amniotic fluid and IUGR. As the placenta is the cause, pre-eclampsia will resolve after delivery.

Symptoms of pre-eclampsia include headache, swelling, and belly pain. Any blood pressure of 140/90 or higher should raise suspicion. (A normal blood pressure in pregnancy is 120/80 or less.)

Most women with mild pre-eclampsia will be managed with bed rest and close monitoring. The chance of getting to 37 weeks is very good if the condition does not become severe. Severe pre-eclampsia requires delivery; however, in some cases your doctors may try to stabilize your health for 48 hours and give you steroids to improve your baby's survival and outcome. Delaying delivery in severe pre-eclampsia requires obstetricians with advanced training. If you have severe pre-eclampsia, you will also receive **magnesium sulfate,** which helps to prevent seizures. The dose of *magnesium sulfate* to prevent seizures is different from the dose to protect against cerebral palsy.

High Blood Pressure

Not all high blood pressure in pregnancy is pre-eclampsia, although it's still concerning as it may affect your placenta, increasing your risk of growth restriction (IUGR) and abruption (bleeding behind the placenta). High blood pressure can also damage your organs, such as kidneys, heart, brain, and eyes, and increases your risk of pre-eclampsia.

Unlike pre-eclampsia, high blood pressure can often be treated with medications. Premature delivery may be recommended if your blood pressure is difficult to control or there are signs that you or your baby may be having problems.

Abruption

Placental abruption is a condition in which some of the placenta separates from the wall of your uterus, causing the underlying surface of the uterus to bleed. The blood may clot and stay trapped behind the placenta or may leak out, causing vaginal bleeding.

Abruption is the most common cause of bleeding in the second and third trimesters.

Causes include high blood pressure, infection, smoking, and PPROM. Physical trauma to the belly and cocaine use can also cause the placenta to separate.

There are no good tests for abruption; ultrasound can only detect a very large blood clot, so it rarely helps. Abruption should be considered when any of the following are present: preterm contractions, PPROM, a tender belly, or vaginal bleeding. If you have a suspected abruption, you will be admitted to the hospital; both mother and baby will need close monitoring to make sure blood loss is not excessive and to ensure that the baby is getting enough oxygen. Close monitoring for signs of labor is also essential. If you have a lot of bleeding you may need a blood transfusion.

Abruption can lead to premature delivery in several ways:

- **Indicated delivery** due to excessive blood loss for you or your baby.
- **Preterm labor,** as blood irritates the uterus, triggering contractions.
- **PPROM,** because bleeding weakens the membranes inside the uterus.
- **IUGR** due to a damaged placenta.

Placenta Previa

In this condition, the placenta is too low in the uterus and covers your cervix. As your cervix starts to soften and open in the third trimester, the placenta can detach, causing bleeding. This precludes a vaginal delivery, not only because the placenta is physically blocking the cervix, but also because labor can produce catastrophic bleeding.

Placenta previa may be due to scarring in the uterus (typically due to a previous C-section), a large placenta, or an abnormally shaped uterus. It should be suspected if you have vaginal bleeding in the second or third trimesters; however, not all women have bleeding. The diagnosis of placenta previa is made by ultrasound.

Bed rest is recommended to keep your uterus as quiet as possible. Any bleeding must be evaluated immediately. If you have persistent bleeding, you may need to be hospitalized. Heavy bleeding may require a blood transfusion or an emergency C-section if the blood loss is affecting you or your baby. As the risk of a premature delivery is high, most women re-

Soon after I was admitted to the hospital, my secretary, Gail, left me with a copy of Dan Brown's *The Da Vinci Code*. I thought she was crazy—there was no way I would be able to concentrate enough to read. But one does not argue with Gail. "What else do you have to do?" she said, rolling her eyes at me and dropping the book on my bedside table.

The *Mona Lisa* stared at me from the cover as if she were Gail's personal emissary. After a day I gave in, and within a few minutes I was transported to France. Those hours when I was lost in the pages were incredibly therapeutic, a wonderful break from the emotional seesaw of stress and boredom.

By the time the boys delivered, I had read 20 books, become a Sudoku master, watched 40 or so episodes of *Law and Order* (it is always on), and become hooked on several reality shows. I developed a schedule around these events, ending at 11 PM when my husband called and we talked about our respective days as if we were sitting at the dinner table.

We are all creatures of habit and routines, and it's overwhelming when that basic core is breached. Re-establishing a routine, no matter how ordinary the activities, and sticking to it like a job helped me maintain a small amount of certainty when everything else was an unknown.

ceive steroids between 24 and 30 weeks (the exact timing will vary from patient to patient) to help the baby's lungs and other organ systems to mature. If your pregnancy is otherwise uncomplicated, a C-section will be performed at 36 weeks because the risk of labor starts to increase at 37 weeks.

Antiphospholipid Antibody Syndrome

This syndrome, a disease of the immune system, results in the production of abnormal antibodies. Antibodies normally fight infection, but these abnormal ones cause blood to clot inappropriately. During pregnancy the risk of blood clots is already elevated, and antiphospholipid antibody syndrome increases your risk even further. Blood clots can lead to serious lung problems and even stroke for the mother. Damage to the placenta from blood clots can lead to IUGR and pre-eclampsia.

Antiphospholipid antibody syndrome is treated with blood thin-
ners, close monitoring for pre-eclampsia and blood clots, and frequent
ultrasounds to screen for IUGR. A specialist should be involved, but with
the appropriate therapy, more than 75 percent of women will have a successful pregnancy.

3

Multiple Pregnancy

When you're pregnant with two or more babies, it's called a multiple pregnancy. The risk of a premature delivery is dramatically increased: In the United States 3 percent of all births are multiples, yet almost 20 percent of premature babies are multiples. In fact, for every family who delivers their twins after 35 weeks, there is another family who delivers before 35 weeks (Table 1). The risk of almost every condition that can lead to premature delivery is increased with multiples, and these problems often occur earlier in the pregnancy. For example, the risk of pre-eclampsia is more than doubled, and the risk of abruption is increased eightfold. It's a hard reality, but prematurity is just the price of business with multiples.

TABLE 1: Multiple Gestation, Prematurity, and Outcome (Adapted from American Congress of Obstetricians and Gynecologists Practice Bulletin #56, Multiple Gestation, 2004)

	Average gestational age at delivery	Percent needing NICU admission	Babies with major disability	Average length NICU stay
Twins	35 weeks	25%	3%	18 days
Triplets	32 weeks	75%	20%	30 days
Quadruplets	30 weeks	100%	50%	58 days

I see the rare family on TV with successful quadruplets, quintuplets, or even sextuplets and I have to admit these stories stir difficult emotions. Negative thoughts race through my mind, such as, *She got six babies to 30 weeks and I couldn't even do three?* It's easy to let these stories percolate in your head, and after a while you start to think that you must have done something wrong, because you don't read a lot of stories about the families who are sitting in neonatal intensive units wondering if their premature multiples will be able to go to school one day, or if they will ever come home.

After a few minutes of gratuitous moping, I pull myself together and remind myself that those families who take home six or eight babies won the lottery. And then I shake my head and move on with my life.

Two-thirds of twins and most higher-order multiples (triplets, quadruplets, and so on) are fraternal, meaning the babies are siblings, each from a unique egg and sperm, that just happen to be sharing the uterus. The remaining one-third of twins are identical, meaning they come from one fertilized egg (one egg and one sperm) that splits into two identical copies. The odds of identical triplets are about one in a million, and they are astronomical for identical quadruplets and quintuplets.

The most important point about a multiple pregnancy is the number of amniotic sacs and membranes. A baby grows in an amniotic sac made of two membranes, called a **chorion** (outer membrane) and an **amnion** (inner membrane, closest to the baby). Fraternal twins always have two separate sacs, with one chorion and one amnion for each baby, so they are also called **dichorionic/diamnionic twins.** For identical twins, the number of membrane layers is dictated by how soon the fertilized egg splits. If the split is within two days after fertilization, each baby will develop in its own two-layer sac, just as dichorionic/diamnionic twins do. A division of the fertilized egg on days three through eight leaves one chorion (the outer membrane) and two inner amnions. Each baby is still in an individual sac separated only by its amnions (**monochorionic/ diamnionic twins**). A split on days nine to eleven leaves only one set of membranes, called **monochorionic/monoamnionic.** This means that both twins are developing in the same sac, without any dividing membranes.

The best analogy is double bagging groceries where the chorion is the outer bag and the amnion is the inner bag. Imagine you have two tomatoes. You double bag each tomato and then grab both bags at the neck; the tomatoes are each separated from the outside world by two bags and they are separated from each other by four layers. This is dichorionic/diamnionic. Now put each tomato in an individual bag and put both of these two bags in one large bag. The tomatoes are still separated from the outside world by two layers, but are now separated from each other by only two layers. This is analogous to monochorionic/diamnionic. Now double bag the two tomatoes together: This is monochorionic and monoamnionic. The tomatoes are still separated from the environment by two layers, but they are not separated from each other at all.

A first-trimester ultrasound is the best way to identify the membrane situation. As we've seen, the membrane separating diamnionic/dichorionic twins is actually composed of four layers, so it appears thicker on ultrasound. Diamnionic/monochorionic twins only have two layers, so the membrane is much thinner. If no separating membrane is detected, the pregnancy is monochorionic/monoamnionic.

Nutrition

Paying attention to nutritional requirements in a multiple pregnancy improves outcome. Women who see a dietician regularly, closely monitor their nutritional status, follow an individualized dietary plan, and take additional supplements are less likely to deliver prematurely.

The first thing to think about is calories—more babies mean you need more energy. During a singleton pregnancy the average woman needs between 2,300 and 2,800 calories a day (depending on height, activity, and age) and should gain 25 to 35 pounds. Twins need an additional 1,000 calories a day, and higher-order multiples need even more (Table 2).

TABLE 2: Average Calorie Requirements and Weight Gain for Single and Multiple Gestations

	Calories	By 20 weeks	By 28 weeks	Total
Singleton	2,500	12 lbs	20 lbs	25–35 lbs
Twins	3,500	25 lbs	38 lbs	40–56 lbs
Triplets	4,000	35 lbs	54 lbs	58–75 lbs
Quadruplets	4,500	45 lbs	65 lbs	70–80 lbs

The calories should be broken down as follows:

- 20 percent protein
- 40 percent carbohydrates
- 40 percent fat

Ask to meet with a dietician to make sure you are meeting your nutritional needs. While you are waiting, record what you are eating. (The nutritional content of almost every food is available on the labeling or on the Internet.)

With multiples it's difficult, even if you're eating very well, to get enough vitamins, so discuss the following supplements with your OB/GYN:

- **A prenatal vitamin.** In the first trimester, take one a day and start taking two a day in the second trimester.
- **A multivitamin** with 333 mg of calcium, 133 mg of magnesium, and 5 mg of zinc. Take nine tablets divided into three doses throughout the day (basically an extra 3,000 mg a day of calcium, 1,200 mg a day of magnesium, and 45 mg a day of zinc).

Causes of Prematurity
Specific to Multiples

Twin-to-Twin Transfusion Syndrome

When there is one outer sac and two inner sacs (monochorionic/diamnionic pregnancy), there are two placentas, but they remain connected by blood vessels. This connection can allow twins to exchange a small amount of blood with each other. Normally this is balanced, and since the babies have an identical blood type, a small amount of blood traveling back and forth does no harm. Twin-to-twin transfusion syndrome, or TTS, occurs when the placental connection is unbalanced, with one baby always donating and the other always on the receiving end. The risk of this occurring in a monochorionic/diamnionic pregnancy is between 5 percent and 17 percent.

The baby who donates the blood (the donor twin) gets weak and dehydrated, and may even stop growing. The baby on the receiving end (the recipient twin) swells from the blood (this is called **hydrops**) and produces more and more amniotic fluid (called **polyhydramnios**) in an attempt to get rid of the surplus blood. Both babies are at risk for brain injury, heart problems, and even death. It's impossible to predict whether monochorionic/diamnionic twins will develop TTS or how serious it will get, so close observation with ultrasound, especially between 18 and 24 weeks (when severe TTS is most likely to develop) is recommended. TTS is one of the reasons it's important to know the type of membrane, because TTS is unique to monochorionic/diamnionic pregnancies.

In addition to ultrasound, other tests can help with the diagnosis of TTS including:

- **A Doppler test,** which is a special ultrasound that detects abnormal blood flow.
- **An MRI** (magnetic resonance imaging), a special scan that produces very detailed images of the placenta, blood vessels, and membranes without harmful X-rays.

How TTS is managed depends on gestational age, the stage of the condition, and the health of your babies. The stage is determined by ultrasound:

- **Stage 1: Abnormal amount of amniotic fluid around one baby.**
- **Stage 2: Lack of urine in the bladder of the donor twin (a sign of dehydration).**
- **Stage 3: Abnormal blood flow detected with Doppler ultrasound.**
- **Stage 4: Swelling of the recipient twin.**
- **Stage 5: Death of one baby.**

TTS should never be taken lightly. If it progresses to stage 2 or beyond and is left untreated, the risk of one baby dying is very high; if one baby passes away, the risk to the surviving baby in the next 24 hours is significant. Therapy for TTS includes:

- **Amniocentesis** to remove excess amniotic fluid from the recipient twin. This relieves pressure, temporarily improving circulation for the donor. The fluid will continue to re-accumulate as long as the abnormal blood flow is present.
- **Surgery to interrupt the connection between the blood vessels.** While technically challenging, surgery offers the best chance for survival and the lowest risk of heart and brain complications.
- **Septostomy,** which is a puncture of the membranes between the twins, evenly distributing the amniotic fluid around each baby.
- **Premature delivery.**

Babies with TTS are also at risk for spontaneous premature delivery. The increased fluid and corrective procedures (like amniocentesis or surgery to interrupt the blood vessels) can cause preterm premature rupture of membranes (PPROM) or premature labor.

Monoamnionic Twins

Monoamnionic twins are in the same sac without a dividing membrane. The biggest risk is tangling or even knotting of the umbilical cords, which affects the flow of oxygen. This is called a **cord accident,** and the consequences include brain injury, poor growth, and even stillbirth. Without proper obstetrical care, the risk of both twins dying can be as high as 50 percent; *however,* with the right management, that risk drops to less than 10 percent.

Special care of monoamnionic twins involves:

- **Ultrasounds every four weeks for growth.**
- **Heart rate monitoring starting between 24 and 28 weeks.** There is no consensus among experts regarding the optimal frequency of monitoring; the protocols range anywhere from three times a week to three times a day.
- **Planned delivery by C-section between 32 and 36 weeks.** Once your babies are 32 weeks, the risk of a cord accident may start outweighing the risks of prematurity. There is no consensus for the optimal timing of delivery. Monoamnionic twins should not deliver vaginally.

Discordant Growth

When one twin has intrauterine growth restriction (IUGR, see chapter 3) and is at least 20 to 25 percent smaller than the other, the condition is called discordant growth. While any condition that can cause IUGR may be involved, the most common causes are:

- **Impaired placental health,** when crowding from multiple placentas affects the transport of oxygen and other nutrients.
- **Abnormal connection of the umbilical cord to the placenta.**
- **Twin-to-twin transfusion syndrome.**

If the smaller twin is having significant problems, parents may be faced with the heart-wrenching decision of having an early delivery for the sake of the smaller, sick baby. While this may save the life of the smaller twin, it also exposes the healthier, larger baby to the risks of prematurity. Because these kinds of management decisions are very complex, the best advice is to make sure you are under the care of an experienced perinatologist with input from a neonatologist.

Reduction

If you are pregnant with higher-order multiples (triplets, quadruplets, and so on), your OB/GYN will discuss selective reduction. This is a procedure to reduce the number of babies to improve the chances of survival and reduce the risk of severe disability for the remaining babies.

The procedure is performed between 11 and 12 weeks. Reduction is not an option for babies in a monochorionic pregnancy (fertilized egg that splits on day three or later), who are connected with each other via their shared circulation.

The average gestational age of triplets is 32 weeks, and the odds that all three babies will survive to come home from the hospital are 87 percent. Reduction to twins increases the average gestational age to 36 weeks

> We had barely accepted that I was pregnant when my doctor asked if we wanted to consider a reduction. The investment to get here and then the irony of the decisions you have to make to stay!
>
> It's strange how these things work, but considering whether to have the reduction or not was a gift. Once we reached our decision not to reduce, my husband and I vowed there would be no looking back and no what-ifs, because you can quickly drive yourself mad wondering what might have been. We all have difficult choices, but that's the nature of parenting. For some of us these choices start sooner than they should, and you just have to do the best you can with the information you have. That's all you can ask of yourself.

and the odds that both of these babies come home from the hospital is 88 percent. Most obstetricians do not recommend or dissuade parents from reducing with triplets, they simply present the information.

Reduction has a greater impact for quadruplets and other higher-order multiples. With reduction, the risk of an extremely premature delivery (delivering before 28 weeks) drops significantly. A mother's risk of complications is also lower with reduction. This should not be dismissed, as high-order multiples are an incredible health strain, and the risk of a poor outcome for mom is significantly increased. Most obstetricians recommend that parents consider reduction with quadruplets and other higher-order multiples.

The Delivery

When planning for your delivery of multiples, your OB/GYN will consider many factors, including your health, the position of your babies (head down or breech), estimated birth weights, and whether one or both of your babies are growth restricted (IUGR). A vaginal delivery will take place in an operating room in case the medical situation changes and a C-section is needed.

Both of your babies will be closely monitored during labor and delivery. After your first baby delivers, an ultrasound will be used to confirm the position of your second baby. If she is head down, then your second labor will proceed just as the first one. If your second baby is breech, a vaginal delivery may or may not be possible—it will depend on many individual factors.

With multiples there are certain situations when a vaginal delivery is not recommended:
- **The presence of severe IUGR (growth restriction)** in one or both babies.
- **Your first baby is breech.**
- **Your twins are in the same sac** (no dividing membrane).
- **You are pregnant with triplets or other high-order multiples.**

Interval Delivery

Premature labor can stop after delivery of the first baby, although it's uncommon. In most cases, labor re-starts within 48 hours; however, there is a small chance the delivery of the remaining babies may be delayed by a week or more. This is called an interval delivery. This delay, or interval of time, has the biggest potential impact for babies who are between 22 and 26 weeks.

The management of an interval delivery is similar to the management of preterm premature rupture of membranes (see chapter 5): antibiotics, steroids, and close observation for infection. Tocolytics to stop labor may also be indicated for 48 hours to allow time to administer the steroids. Some doctors may also recommend a stitch to tighten the cervix.

4

Your Delivery

Preparing for your premature delivery is difficult because there are so many variables. How the events unfold depends on factors such as gestational age, your health, your baby's health, and the reason for your delivery.

Some basic ways that a premature delivery differs from one at term include:

- **The need to closely monitor your baby's heartbeat,** because a premature baby may be less capable of handling the physical stress of labor and delivery.
- **A greater chance of an induction.**
- **An increased likelihood of a C-section.**

There's also the emotional aspect of your delivery. Having a baby at term under the most uncomplicated of circumstances is stressful. When your baby is premature, you have the added worry of your baby's prognosis. Also, you may be less prepared for your delivery. The time sequence from recognizing that you may deliver prematurely to delivery can be very short. You may not have processed the idea or completed childbirth classes. In addition, you could be feeling unwell, either from a medical condition or as a side effect of medications. Some mothers are also mentally exhausted from the lengthy process of hospital admission.

When my boys were about three years old, I was having lunch with a friend who began to tell me about the horrors of her birth experience. She felt her birth plan was ignored. She didn't get to labor in a tub. She had to be monitored, so she couldn't walk. She felt as if the doctors forced her to have an epidural. And she didn't like the room or the meals, for that matter. So I asked how her baby was doing. "Oh, she's fine," and then my friend started on again about the horrors of a modern labor and delivery suite.

I couldn't believe it. A full-term, healthy baby and she was upset? I sat on my hands, because my first reaction was to slap her. I was angry that she could not see how lucky she was, and jealous because I would have given everything to have my boys at term.

Pregnancy and delivery are two pieces of a puzzle, and for closure the pieces must fit. Everyone's vision for her birth experience is different. For some it is laboring in a tub at moonlight and for others it might be an epidural at the first contraction. However, no one's birth plan is a premature delivery, so listening to someone talk negatively about their full-term delivery, for me, was like watching someone wave that missing puzzle piece just out of my reach.

It's been helpful to acknowledge that missing my desired birth experience has had a profound effect. For the record: It was C-section at term. I can't change it, but accepting this as a loss has been helpful, and allowed me to move on.

Anesthesia

Many women need pain relief (anesthesia) for their vaginal delivery; with a C-section it is essential. Labor is painful, and some women with medically indicated premature deliveries (such as pre-eclampsia) need an induction to bring on labor, which can mean many hours or even a day or two of painful contractions. While a support person can help you to cope, there are fewer options for natural pain relief, such as walking or taking a shower, because your baby will almost certainly need continuous heart-rate monitoring. You may also be feeling too unwell to fully participate.

Intravenous painkillers, such as *morphine* or *fentanyl*, can be used to treat the pain of contractions; however, they are not always an option. If they are given too close to delivery, they can depress your baby's drive to breathe. The best medical options for pain control are an *epidural* or a *spinal*. With both of these procedures, an anesthetic (a substance that numbs the nerves and tissues) is injected around the spinal cord. With a spinal the medication is placed directly into the fluid that surrounds the spinal cord; with an epidural the medication is administered into the area outside this fluid sac but very close to the spinal cord. The anesthetic does not enter the bloodstream, so there will be no effect on your baby's breathing. An epidural is the best medical option for a vaginal delivery because it can be maintained over several days if needed and the dose can be reduced when it's time to deliver, so you can be a more effective pusher. The dose can also be increased so you can have a C-section. A spinal anesthetic will last for about an hour, so it is the best option if the only plan for your delivery is a C-section. With both an epidural and a spinal, you will not be able to tell if your bladder is full, so a bladder catheter will be needed.

Epidurals and spinals are very safe. The risk of a complication with a severe and lasting effect is less than 0.1 percent. The biggest concern is bleeding around the spinal cord. For most women this risk is very low, because the injured blood vessels form clots almost immediately, which stop the bleeding. However, this protective mechanism may not work if you have a bleeding problem, so every woman must have a blood test to check the level of platelets (a major component of blood clotting) in her blood beforehand. Low platelet levels are most common with preeclampsia. (See chapter 2.)

The biggest risk for your baby from placement of an epidural or spinal anesthetic is a drop in your blood pressure, which can lower the baby's heart rate. This is usually preventable with careful monitoring and extra fluid in the IV before the procedure.

Your Delivery

Vaginal

You may labor spontaneously or require an induction. There are two medications used to induce labor: *oxytocin*, which is administered by IV, and *prostaglandins* (such as *misoprostol, Cervidil,* or *Prepidil*), which are administered vaginally. *Oxytocin* and *prostaglandins* cannot be given together, although they can be used sequentially.

During labor and delivery your baby's heart rate will be closely monitored to ensure she is tolerating the physical stress. The delivery itself may happen in a labor room or in an operating room if your OB/GYN is concerned that a C-section may ultimately be required.

Having your partner or a doula with you may help. A support person is comforting, can help you cope, and, from a practical standpoint, can be useful to keep track of everything that is happening.

Regardless of how your labor starts, once your cervix reaches 4 to 5 cm dilation, things usually progress very quickly; many premature babies can fit through a cervix that is not fully dilated (less than 10 cm), and a smaller baby requires less pushing. It's hard to imagine a premature baby, many weighing less than 1,000 g (2 lbs, 3 oz), withstanding a vaginal delivery, but studies have not shown that a C-section is safer.

As soon as your baby is delivered, your doctor will clamp the umbilical cord and immediately hand your baby to the pediatrics team. The next step is your placenta, which should deliver within 30 minutes. Problems with delivering the placenta are more common after a preterm delivery—a premature placenta may not separate completely from the uterus, and medical problems such as pre-eclampsia and infection can contribute to excessive bleeding. There are procedures your OB/GYN can perform to remove the placenta or stop the bleeding if necessary.

Your bottom may be swollen and sore after a vaginal delivery, more so if you have a tear, episiotomy, or hemorrhoids. Fortunately, this area of the body heals quickly. The three most important things to speed recovery are:

- **Ice** to reduce swelling and pain. The sooner, the better.
- **Pain medicine,** usually *ibuprofen*-like medication, although some women may require something stronger.
- **Preventing constipation.** Passing hard, large stools is very painful, especially if you have stitches or hemorrhoids. Keeping your stool

soft with a medication called *ducosate sodium* (*Colace*) can help. Opioid medications, such as *Vicodin* or *Percocet*, are constipating, so if you need one of these drugs to help with your pain, it's wise to also take a laxative.

Cesarean Section

About 50 percent of premature deliveries are C-section. The most common reasons:

- **Not enough time to induce labor.** You or your baby may have urgent medical conditions such that waiting even a few hours could be dangerous.
- **Your baby is significantly growth restricted** (intrauterine growth restriction, or IUGR) and may not be receiving enough oxygen and nutrition to cope with the physical stress of labor.
- **Your baby is breech** (bottom down). Premature babies are more likely to be in the breech position.

A C-section happens in an operating room. The first step is to make sure you have adequate anesthesia for the surgery. An epidural or spinal is the safest choice for both mom and baby, and there is the added benefit of being able to stay awake to see your baby. However, there are times when a general anesthetic (going to sleep) is needed. The most common reasons are:

- **An emergency,** because a general anesthetic is generally faster. In some situations, even a few minutes may have an impact on your baby's outcome.
- **Medical conditions such as those that affect blood clotting,** making it unsafe to have an epidural or spinal.
- **Technical difficulties** placing the epidural or spinal.

If you need a general anesthetic, the anesthesiologist will choose medications that are safest for your baby; however, many babies will be sleepy when they are born. The pediatrics team knows how to provide support until these effects wear off.

With an epidural or spinal, your support person is generally allowed to come into the operating room and sit with you at the head of the operating table. They can talk with you, hold your hand, or stroke your hair. However, in most hospitals if you need a general anesthetic, your support person cannot come into the operating room.

Most C-sections are performed with a horizontal incision just above the pubic hair (this is often called a bikini-line incision); however, there are some situations in which your doctor may feel an up-and-down incision (also called a midline or vertical incision) is the safer option. An uncomplicated C-section takes about 45 minutes, but there is extra time both before and after for setting up and taking down equipment. Your baby is delivered within the first few minutes, and then removing the placenta and repairing your uterus and tissues occupies the rest of the time. If you're awake, you will feel pressure (sometimes a lot) and tugging or pulling, but it shouldn't hurt. If you're in any pain or feeling anxious, the anesthesiologist can help in many ways, from reassuring you to providing medications for pain or anxiety.

You will need close observation after a C-section. Your nurse will monitor your blood pressure, heart rate, and oxygen levels and will press on your belly to ensure that your uterus is contracting enough to stop bleeding. They'll also look at the bandage over your incision and your pad to check on your bleeding. Your nurse may massage your belly, stimulating your uterus to contract more and squeezing the blood vessels shut. With an epidural or a spinal, you will be in the recovery area until the anesthetic has worn off and you can move your legs. If you received a general anesthetic, you will be in recovery until you are awake enough to cough and clear your own airways. Your nurse will also administer pain medications or medications for nausea and vomiting as needed. This immediate recovery from a C-section generally takes one to two hours, but it could be longer. Everyone understands that you are anxious to see your baby; however, a C-section is major surgery and close monitoring is essential.

It is normal to need pain medication after a C-section. Surgery hurts, and worrying about your baby makes pain worse. Pain can keep you from walking (important for your recovery) and from interacting with your baby, and it makes it harder to process what is happening in the NICU. In addition to *ibuprofen,* most women need an opioid medication for at least a few days.

Three days after my C-section I was still in incredible pain. My body was deconditioned from prolonged bed rest, and the infection in my bloodstream still wracked my body with sweats that soaked my sheets and chills that made me shake so hard my muscles ached. I didn't think I could take any more.

One of the nurses announced that I was going to have a shower. I thought she was crazy. I could barely stand up, and getting to the bathroom was monumental effort that required an hour of recovery. But she dismissed my fears with a wave of her hand. "You'll feel better," she said, more like an order than a statement.

She got me out of bed and held my arm while I shuffled to the bathroom. And then, just as if I were her baby, she undressed me, sat me on a seat in the shower, and proceeded to wash me from head to toe. As the water ran over me I started to cry, but she just kept talking away and washing. By the time she dressed me and put me back to bed, in clean sheets, I felt better than I had in a long while. But it wasn't just the shower. Having someone devote that much care to you is the best kind of healing.

PART TWO

Your Premature Baby and the Hospital

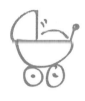

5

The First Few Days

It's hard enough adjusting to the stresses of parenthood, never mind this strange new world of prematurity. If you're unable to hold your baby, that will only add to your feelings of helplessness and worry. Understanding what is happening in these first few days—where your baby is going, who is looking after her, and the medical challenges—are the first steps in orienting yourself and regaining some sense of control.

Resuscitation

The first minutes after your baby is born are devoted to resuscitation, which is the immediate medical care after birth. Once your baby's medical condition is stable, she will be transported to an intensive care nursery where a more thorough assessment is performed. If your baby is 35 or 36 weeks, medically stable, and there are no concerns about infection, she may not need specialized care and may be able to stay in your room.

Two or three skilled members of the neonatal team will perform the resuscitation. It might look and sound like mayhem, but the team is working together using terminology they all understand. The team will proceed through three steps in very rapid succession, with the main goal of making sure your baby is getting enough oxygen into her lungs and that her heart is delivering the oxygen to her tissues. The three steps are:

1. **Initial stabilization and evaluation.** Immediately after delivery your baby will be handed to a member of the resuscitation team and placed on a radiant warmer, which is an elevated platform with an overhead heat lamp. As your baby is being dried, monitors will be placed to record oxygen level, heart rate, and temperature. She will get a knit cap to prevent heat loss, and some very tiny babies are immediately wrapped in plastic up to the neck to trap in body heat. Fluid will be suctioned from the mouth, nose, and lungs with a thin tube, and oxygen will be administered.

2. **Assessment of breathing and oxygen levels.** A healthy newborn takes 40 to 60 breaths per minute. The ideal oxygen level for a premature baby is controversial; however, most doctors want to keep the levels above 85 percent. If needed, supplemental oxygen may be given by a face mask. Oxygen may also be pushed into the lungs under pressure. (See chapter 6 for a description of methods.) Some babies will need an **endotracheal tube** (breathing tube), which is a tube through the mouth into the windpipe to help the lungs function more effectively. This also allows the lungs to be suctioned to remove any fluid. Surfactant, a medication that helps stabilize premature air sacs, may be administered into the breathing tube so it can spread to the lungs.

3. **Heart rate and circulation.** Treatment is needed if your baby's heart rate is less than 100 beats per minute (bpm). A slow heart rate may improve with additional oxygen, but IV fluids may also be needed. If the heart rate drops below 60 bpm, **cardiopulmonary resuscitation** (CPR or chest compressions) is necessary to push blood from the heart to the rest of the body while other therapies are started.

Your baby will be assigned an Apgar score during her resuscitation. The Apgar score is an indication of how much resuscitation your baby needed after birth. It has five components: heart rate, respiratory effort, muscle tone, reflex irritability (response to stimulation), and color. Each is given a score of 0, 1, or 2. The score is reported at one and five minutes after birth; a five-minute score of 7 to 10 is considered normal for a baby born at term. If the Apgar score is less than 7 at five minutes, the scoring is repeated every five minutes up to 20 minutes, so many preemies end up with five scores. Do not get caught up in the Apgar score—a premature baby is *expected* to have lower scores, because muscle tone, color, and reflex irritability (three of the five scoring tools) vary by gestational age.

Transfer

Once your baby is stabilized, she will be transported to the nursery in an incubator, which is an enclosed, highly specialized box that keeps your baby warm and protected from noise, drafts, infection, and excessive handling. Incubators are often called "isolettes," but Isolette is actually the brand name of an incubator (like Kleenex for facial tissue). Some babies who are only a few weeks premature and medically stable may be swaddled in a blanket and carried to the nursery by a nurse. Many late preterm babies (35 to 36 weeks) will not need an intensive care setting and, after the initial assessment, will be able to stay with you and go to a regular nursery.

You will still be recovering when your baby is transferred, but if your baby is stable, the team will stop to give you and your partner a brief update and a glimpse. They know you are desperate for news and to see your baby, but the number one priority is getting your baby stabilized. Your partner may be invited along to the intensive care unit or may be asked to wait behind in the delivery room. This does not necessarily mean your baby is sicker than others; the policies vary from one hospital to another. A doctor or nurse practitioner will come back and provide information once your baby's situation is stable.

Where Is My Baby Going?

There are three types of nurseries ranked by the intensity of care they can provide:

I was still being sewn up from my C-section when the neonatal team left with Oliver. He was so sick they couldn't even pause to take footprints for his birth certificate. My surgery was over, but I was still on the operating table when the team stopped by with Victor. The nurse practitioner lifted him out of the incubator, attached to what seemed like a hundred tubes. I remember begging, "No, don't. Put him back, please, just take him to the NICU." I was terrified that those few seconds out of his fortress on wheels would be his demise. But she smiled and replied, "He'll be okay and you will remember this forever." And she was right. The fraction of a second when I felt his little fingers and knew that he was real were amazing. The tubes, wires, monitors, and noise seemed to slip away, and all I could see was his tiny little preciousness.

- **A level 1** nursery, also called a newborn nursery, is a nursery for healthy babies who can maintain their body temperature and do not require special monitoring, oxygen, or IVs. Many babies born between 35 and 37 weeks will be able to go to a level 1 nursery.
- **A level 2 nursery** is a neonatal intensive care unit (NICU) that offers advanced medical and nursing care and generally accepts babies 32 weeks or older. Babies in level 2 nurseries can receive oxygen, be fed by a tube, and take medications and nourishment intravenously.
- **A level 3 nursery** is an NICU that is equipped to care for the sickest and the smallest babies (although some level 3 units are not able to handle babies under 1,000 g [2 lbs, 3 oz] and some are not equipped to provide open-heart surgery). Most hospitals with a level 3 nursery do not have a separate level 2, so the level 3 NICU cares for every baby that cannot go to a level 1 nursery. Babies that require the help of a machine to breathe (also called mechanical ventilation) for more than 24 hours should be in a level 3 NICU.

Who Is Caring for My Baby?

Knowing who will be involved in your baby's care and their role is very helpful, especially as you may be working with these people for weeks or even months. Your baby's health care team may include some or all of these professionals:

- **Neonatologist.** A doctor who has completed six years of training (three years of general pediatrics and three years in the care of premature babies and the critical care needs of newborns). They are captains of the ship in a level 2 or 3 nursery; they make decisions, order medications, and perform procedures. They are responsible for all the care provided by the nurse practitioners, and in training hospitals they are also responsible for the care provided by the pediatric residents.
- **Neonatology fellow.** A pediatrician enrolled in a three-year training program learning to be a neonatologist.
- **Pediatrician.** A doctor who has completed three years of training (called residency) in the care of children. A pediatrician may run a level 2 nursery or work in an NICU as part of the team.
- **Pediatrics resident.** A doctor in residency learning to become a pediatrician.
- **Pediatrics intern.** A first-year pediatrics resident.
- **Nurse practitioner (NP).** A nurse who has completed advanced education and training. An NP works closely with the neonatologist or pediatrician and functions like a physician, ordering tests and medications.
- **Nurse.** A nurse manages your baby's daily needs, administers medications, and works much of the equipment. Your baby's primary nurse physically interacts with you and your baby the most.
- **Respiratory therapist (RT).** A health care practitioner who specializes in the assessment and treatment of respiratory tract disorders (problems with lungs and airways). RTs can **intubate** (insert

a breathing tube) and are skilled at working the complex equipment and oxygen supplies needed to support breathing.

- **Physical therapist (PT)** and **occupational therapist (OT).** Medical professionals who specialize in movement, coordination, and the skills we need for everyday living. They work with babies to reduce the impact of prematurity on the nervous system and muscles.
- **Social worker.** A professional who provides families with supportive counseling; connects parents with community, state, and federal resources; and organizes many aspects of discharge home from the hospital.

After my C-section, my nurse wheeled me on a gurney, flat on my back, down the hall to the NICU. Once inside, she expertly maneuvered the labyrinth of equipment until we stopped at Oliver. I could see tiny feet underneath plastic wrap surrounded by a Medusa's nest of hoses, tubes, and wires. It was just too much. My nurse was one step ahead. "You've had enough," she said, as she whisked me to my room. My boys' nurse told me to call anytime from my room if I wanted to check in. She pressed a piece of paper with the number into my hand as I was wheeled away.

Back in my room I started to worry. I wanted to call, but all of sudden I didn't feel like anyone's mom. There were no flowers or balloons in my room. No waiting pile of diapers or layette. No babies. In, fact there was no physical evidence I had even been pregnant, except for that scrap of paper.

I stared at it for a while, afraid to call. When I finally did I blurted out in about two seconds, "This-is-Oliver-and-Victor's-mom-can-I-speak-with-their-nurse?" I felt like a teenager calling for a first date. I don't remember anything she said, but it was so affirming to hear myself say those words out loud. Gradually, like a fire that is slow to start on wet kindling, the concept that I had two little boys ignited. I probably called five times that night, and every time I said I was Oliver and Victor's mom, the fire burned a little brighter, and I finally drifted off to sleep in the early hours of the day.

Seeing Your Baby for the First Time

When you visit the nursery, you will speak with your baby's nurse. He or she will tell you how your baby is doing and show you how you can contribute to her care. You should also speak with the doctor or nurse practitioner and ask them to explain what has happened so far, the immediate challenges, and any planned therapies or tests. You won't get specific long-term predictions, which is difficult. The consequences of a premature birth, even what lies ahead in the next few weeks, will only be known with time.

When you first see your baby she may be on a radiant warmer, in an incubator, or in a crib—it depends on birth weight and immediate medical challenges. Once the initial assessment is complete and your baby can maintain her body temperature (generally around a weight of 1,700 g, or 3 lbs, 12 oz) and is not startled by the everyday sounds of an intensive care unit, she can be in a crib; otherwise she'll be in an incubator. It's common practice to cover the incubator with a blanket or quilt; this helps to reduce light and noise even further.

If your baby is in a level 2 or 3 nursery, she'll have her vital signs closely monitored. Some vital signs are monitored continuously and others at specific intervals. The vital signs that will be monitored include:

- **Oxygen level.** This is monitored with an oxygen saturation probe wrapped around a toe or the bottom of a foot. It shines a light, which reads the oxygen level in the blood. (See chapter 6 for more information.)
- **Heart rate** is monitored with small electrodes that stick to the chest with a mild adhesive gel. The electrodes pick up the electrical signals from the heart.
- **Blood pressure** is checked with a blood pressure cuff; there are very small sizes made specifically for premature babies. How often your baby's blood pressure is checked will depend on her medical condition; however, the minimum is every four hours. Sicker babies may require continuous blood pressure monitoring using a small catheter placed into one of the arteries in the umbilical cord.

- **Temperature** must be checked frequently, as premature babies lose body heat very quickly. It also is important to make sure they are not getting too warm in the incubator. Temperature is monitored continuously with a probe on the skin or checked regularly with a thermometer under the armpit.
- **Respiratory rate** reflects how hard your baby is working to breath. She should be taking fewer than 40 to 60 breaths a minute and they should be even and not strained.
- **Weight** is measured daily. This is important to ensure that your baby is growing appropriately and not retaining fluid. Some incubators have built-in scales, which makes it very easy. Your baby is lifted, the scale is zeroed, and when she is placed back down a digital readout is obtained. This minimizes physical stress, because babies don't need to be disconnected from equipment or moved into the cold outside environment. If there's no built-in scale or if your baby is in a crib, she will be transferred to a scale every day. This is typically not a problem for a baby who is ready to be in an open crib, but it can be stressful for smaller, sicker babies. Every diaper will also be weighed to help keep track of fluid status.
- **Length and head circumference** will be checked with a paper measuring tape once a week. This can be done without moving your baby.

Other equipment and procedures will vary, depending on your baby's gestational age, birth weight, and medical conditions. The most common equipment includes:

- **Protective eyewear** to shield your baby's eyes from the special lights used to treat jaundice.
- **A feeding tube,** which is a thin tube inserted through the nose (**nasogastric,** or NG, tube) or mouth (**orogastric,** or OG, tube) to the stomach. It's used to give breast milk or formula and medications if your baby is still too immature to suck and swallow in a coordinated manner.

- **Oxygen and breathing equipment.** Your baby may need extra oxygen to breathe or may need specialized equipment to help push oxygen into her lungs. (See chapter 6 for more information.)
- **An intravenous (IV)** for medications, fluid, nutrition, or a blood transfusion. (See Table 1.) Traditional IVs in the hand, foot, or scalp can be difficult to place in premature babies, so many babies will have an umbilical catheter, which involves placement of two thin tubes in the umbilical cord—one tube in an **umbilical artery** and the other tube in the **umbilical vein.** The umbilical artery catheter can also be used to measure blood pressure. Another type of IV is a **peripherally inserted central catheter (PICC,** also called a PIC line), which is a long, specialized IV that goes in a larger vein in the arm or leg. Because a PICC is so long, the tip of the catheter ends in a larger vein close to the heart.

TABLE 1: The Different Types of Intravenous (IV)

	Umbilical catheter	Regular IV	PICC
Where	Artery/vein in umbilical cord	Small vein in foot, hand, or scalp	Large vein in arm or leg
When	Within 7 days of birth	Anytime	Anytime
How long	Taken out within 1–2 weeks	Technically 7 days, but often only lasts 1–2 days	Up to 3 weeks
Painful to insert	No	Yes	Yes
Special issues	Infection is a concern	Too small to give all forms of IV nutrition	Infection is a concern

FIGURE 1: Victor and all of his equipment

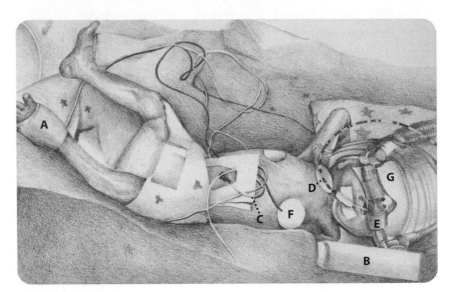

A. oxygen monitor

B. central line (hidden by arm board)

C. umbilical catheter

D. OG tube

E. breathing equipment

F. heart rate monitor

G. eye protection

Assimilating to Life in the Intensive Care Nursery

The metric system is the language of medicine and will be used when weighing and measuring your baby. It is also used for prescribing oxygen and medications. You're probably wondering why you should learn metric on top of everything else? Yes, it's one more thing, and if you are not familiar with grams instead of ounces, it will make everything seem even stranger at first. However, if you learn metric, it will be easier to communicate with your baby's medical team and will help prevent medication errors at home.

The other thing you will not be used to is how the medical team describes the age of a premature baby. There are actually two ways:

- **Unadjusted age** (also called **chronological age**), which is your baby's real age calculated from the day she was born.
- **Adjusted age** (also called **corrected age**), which is calculated from your baby's due date. It makes an allowance for the degree of prematurity. For example, eight weeks after delivery a baby born at 28 weeks has an unadjusted age of two months and an adjusted age of 36 weeks. Adjusted age is typically used in evaluating growth and developmental milestones until two years of age.

FIGURE 2: Unadjusted and adjusted age

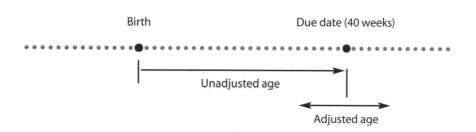

There are a few rules designed to keep the environment in an intensive care nursery protective and productive for every baby:

- **Be vigilant about hand hygiene.** Washing your hands or using hand sanitizer is essential to protect *every* baby in the intensive care unit from infection. Also use hand sanitizer after you touch equipment, other people, or your own mouth and nose before touching your baby.
- **Keep the noise level down.** Premature babies do better in a quiet environment. In addition, you don't want the staff distracted by loud conversations.

- **You may have to leave at change of shift.** Your baby's nurse needs to concentrate on relaying the right information to the next nurse free from distractions. In addition, the amount of medical personnel present during a shift change doubles, so the nursery gets quite crowded. These breaks are the perfect time for you to regroup, take a breather, and even practice some mind-body techniques. (See chapter 15.)

When Can I Hold My Baby?

How soon you can hold your baby depends on her health and her ability to maintain her body temperature. You must also consider that your premature baby's immature nervous system is not equipped to immediately handle our loud, harsh environment—for some babies even touch can sometimes be over-stimulating. If your baby is in a crib, she'll almost certainly be stable enough for you to hold, but your nurse will still monitor your baby to ensure she is tolerating the stimulation.

If your baby is an incubator, then the chances are much lower that you'll be able to hold her right away. However, your baby still needs to be touched—she needs diaper changes, she needs to have her temperature and blood pressure checked, and she needs to be swaddled. Have your nurse show you how to do this, because this is your opportunity to touch your baby on a regular basis. A premature baby is ready to try being held once she can tolerate touch without making her heart rate or oxygen level drop. It's very scary the first time you hold a tiny baby with so many wires and tubes, but the nurse will help you with all the equipment and closely monitor your baby's temperature and other vital signs.

6

Prematurity and the Lungs

The lungs continue to develop until 37 weeks in the pregnancy (term), so every premature baby is at risk for lung problems. The more premature the baby is, the greater the risks can be. The health of your baby's lungs is a major factor in determining her prognosis, both in the hospital and at home.

How Our Lungs Work

The lungs look like upside-down trees (Figure 3) with clusters of balloons instead of leaves (Figure 4). The **trachea** (windpipe) is the trunk and delivers air to the airways, called **bronchi** (larger airways) and **bronchioles** (smaller airways). The balloons at the end of the bronchioles are called **alveoli,** thin-walled sacs that extract oxygen from the air and deliver it to the bloodstream. The alveoli also remove the blood's waste product, carbon dioxide, which is then exhaled.

Lung Development and Prematurity

Prematurity affects the lungs in many ways:

- **Fewer, immature alveoli,** which affects the ability to exchange oxygen for carbon dioxide. During pregnancy, the lungs continue

FIGURE 3: Lungs

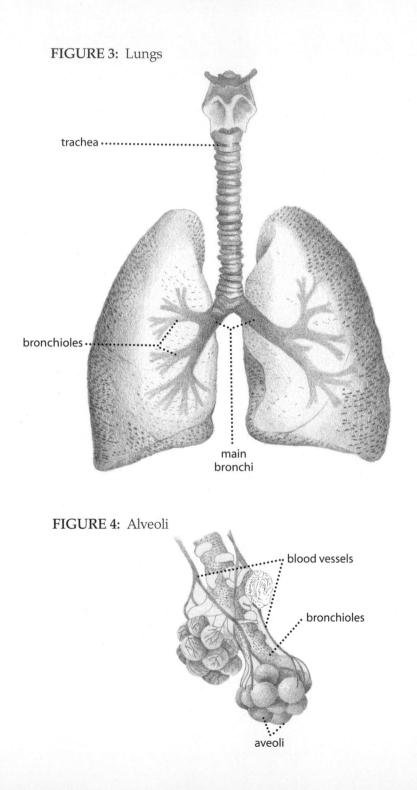

trachea

bronchioles

main
bronchi

FIGURE 4: Alveoli

blood vessels

bronchioles

aveoli

to make alveoli right until delivery. A term baby has 30 to 50 million alveoli, but a premature baby has less, and the more premature the delivery, the fewer the alveoli. These immature alveoli have thicker walls and are less efficient at oxygen transfer. The alveoli are not sufficiently developed to allow breathing until 22 to 26 weeks.

- **Immature blood vessels in the lungs,** which is also gestational age–dependent and affects the ability to transfer oxygen and carbon dioxide.
- **Lack of surfactant,** which is a fatty substance that coats the lining of the alveoli, keeping the tiny balloons from collapsing. Most babies are able to produce enough surfactant at between 30 and 34 weeks.
- **Low amniotic fluid,** which if present affects lung development.
- **Chorioamnionitis,** an infection that can spread from the **amniotic fluid** to the lungs before delivery.

Monitoring Oxygen Levels

Appropriate oxygen levels are important, as more than a few minutes without adequate oxygen can damage the nervous system. However, administering too much oxygen is actually damaging to the lungs and the eyes, so close monitoring is important. The amount of oxygen in the blood is recorded as a percentage called the oxygen saturation. For example, an oxygen saturation of 100 percent means the hemoglobin molecules (the actual oxygen-carrying molecules) in the blood are completely full (saturated) and cannot carry any more oxygen, and a reading of 90 percent means the hemoglobin is carrying 90 percent of its capacity.

The oxygen saturation is monitored continuously with a pulse oximeter (a probe wrapped around the foot or hand). Premature babies have very fragile skin, so the site should be rotated at least every eight hours to prevent skin damage. The normal oxygen saturation is between 95 and 100 percent and typically varies second by second by a few percentage

FIGURE 5: A Normal Oxygen Waveform. Note the regular up-and-down pattern.

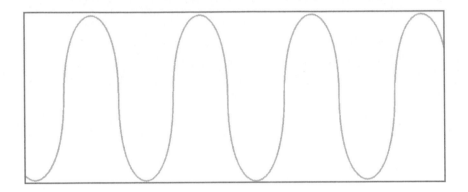

points. Because the monitors are so sensitive, movement can cause the reading to drop sharply for a few seconds, for example, from 96 percent down to 82 percent and then back up to 95 percent.

The oxygen saturation monitors in the NICU also record a waveform. (See Figure 5.) The reading is only accurate if the waveform is an up-and-down pattern that matches the heart rate.

If your baby needs help breathing, most intensive care units will give enough oxygen so the levels fluctuate between a lower saturation of 81 to 85 percent and an upper limit of 90 to 95 percent. If oxygen saturation is boosted to over 95 percent, the risk of serious lung and eye problems increases without improving brain development. It is normal to feel anxious when oxygen levels drop; however, periodic drops below 80 percent will not harm your baby.

The other method of testing the oxygen level is from a blood sample called a blood gas. A blood gas gives more information than an oxygen saturation monitor, but because it involves removing blood, the team will try to limit its use. The blood can be taken from the umbilical artery catheter, but it may also involve a needle stick to withdraw a sample from an artery in the arm.

Oliver and Victor's oxygen saturations were going up and down like a roller coaster. I must have chanted, "Breathe, please breathe," ten thousand times. After a week, I was beside myself. Loss of control mixed with the unknown is the most disempowering of feelings.

I can tell you not to obsess over the monitors, but it's almost impossible. Parents are by nature obsessive over their newborns. It's a normal, protective reflex. Since I couldn't obsess over the car seat or whether the dog licked my baby, I focused on the monitor. When things were going well, the monitors actually blended into the background of life. However, when the alarm went off it was like waving a red flag in front of a bull.

So I spoke with the neonatologist. Even though I had read that oxygen saturation levels in the low 80s were acceptable, I needed to hear it from him. He gave me logical explanations for every one of my questions, and while he could not promise me anything, I was reassured because it was clear that he dealt with this all the time. Having an open line of communication helped me to feel more in control of myself.

Causes of Low Oxygen Levels

There are many reasons your baby may have difficulty breathing:

- **Premature lungs.** The lack of surfactant, weaker muscles, immature alveoli, and underdeveloped blood vessels all make oxygen transfer more difficult.
- **Fatigue.** Some babies will be able to manage for a few days after birth, but then the energy and effort needed to breathe simply become too great.
- **Medical problems** such as infection or bowel issues.
- **Fluid in the lungs,** which makes it harder to transfer oxygen. Fluid can accumulate in the lungs because immature blood vessels are leaky.
- **Patent ductus arteriosus (PDA),** which is a heart condition associated with prematurity. (See chapter 7.)

- **Pneumothorax (collapsed lung).** This happens when one or more alveoli (air sacs) rupture, allowing air to leak out of the lungs into the chest cavity.
- **Pneumonia,** which is infection in the lungs.

Another breathing problem is **apnea,** which is the absence of breathing for more than 20 seconds or a shorter pause that is associated with a drop in the oxygen level or heart rate. Apnea can be divided into two groups:

- **Apnea of prematurity,** when the immature nervous system is unable to trigger a breath. Apnea is common among babies less than 34 weeks at birth and can persist until an adjusted age of 37 weeks, or sometimes longer.
- **Everything else.** Apnea is also an early warning signal for many potentially serious medical conditions. A baby communicates with her body, and one of the best ways to get attention is to stop breathing. Medical conditions that can cause apnea include infection, bowel problems, unstable temperature, low oxygen levels, heart problems, chemical imbalance in the blood, and brain injury.

Clues about the cause of apnea include the pattern (a gradual increase or an abrupt change), the severity, and how easily it responds to therapy. Blood tests and other investigations may be required. The treatment of apnea includes:

- **Stimulation.** Touching can stimulate a breath, but sometimes more vigorous stimulation, such as rubbing the back, is needed.
- **Caffeine** to stimulate the nervous system.
- **Increasing the degree of respiratory support,** meaning more oxygen, more help from machines, or both.
- **Correcting the underlying cause** if one is found.

Respiratory Support

Many premature babies need help with breathing. Because oxygen and some of the equipment can damage the lungs and eyes, the goal is to provide the least amount of support to keep the oxygen levels in the desired range. Every baby is unique, so this requires a lot of fine-tuning. Throughout this process it's not uncommon to have two steps forward and one, or sometimes more, steps backward.

The team will use the oxygen levels and other vital signs like respiratory rate, respiratory effort (how hard a baby appears to be working to breathe), and heart rate to guide the degree of respiratory support.

Supplemental oxygen is given when a baby needs some help with her oxygen levels but can breathe on her own. Room air has 21 percent oxygen, but the oxygen concentration can be increased if needed (even up to 100 percent pure oxygen) to meet your baby's specific needs. Oxygen spreads from areas of high concentration (the airways and air sacs) to areas with less oxygen (the blood); this is analogous to a rock rolling down a hill, traveling from a higher spot to a lower spot. Increasing the concentration of oxygen in the air is like making the hill steeper; more oxygen enters the lung so more gets into the bloodstream. Supplemental oxygen can be given in one of two ways:

- **Nasal prongs (also called nasal cannula),** which are small, soft, plastic tubes that fit in the nostrils. The flow of oxygen can be adjusted from as low as $1/_{32}$ L/min (liters per minute) up to 2 L/min (It can go higher, but 2 L/min is a high flow rate for a baby.) The cannulas are secured with adhesive strips that look like small band-aids.
- **An oxygen hood,** which is a small, clear box filled with oxygen that fits over your baby's head while she is lying in a crib. An oxygen hood is most appropriate for babies close to term who may only need oxygen for a short period of time.

Some babies need help getting oxygen in and out of the lungs. In this situation a machine can help deliver the oxygen to the lungs. The two choices are CPAP, which stands for continuous positive airway pressure, and a ventilator.

- **CPAP** consists of nasal tubes (similar to nasal prongs) or a mask over the nose, both of which force in oxygen-rich air under pressure. The extra pressure helps keep stiff preemie lungs open, reducing the work of breathing. Your baby still has to take the breath (initiate the inhale), but it will be easier. CPAP is like a splint, keeping the airways open; think of CPAP as clearing a path for the rock rolling down the hill. CPAP is less damaging to lungs than a ventilator. The biggest issue is care of the nose, because the skin can get irritated and raw.
- **A ventilator** is a machine that pushes oxygen-rich air into the lungs and removes carbon dioxide. A breathing tube is placed in the trachea (windpipe) and attached via hoses to a machine at the bedside. Going back to the rock and the hill analogy, a ventilator both clears the path and guides the rock down the hill; the degree of force depends on the settings. Ventilator settings are complex and include the oxygen concentration, the number of breaths per minute (respiratory rate), pressure to splint the airways open (called PEEP, or positive end expiratory pressure), and the pressure and the volume of each breath. A ventilator can do all of the work of breathing or can be set to provide some assistance. Ventilators are so sensitive that they can be set to trigger only when a baby starts to take a breath, providing help for that breath only (this is called the assist mode). Some babies get agitated on a ventilator and may need sedation, although the team will try and avoid this, because sedatives reduce the drive to breathe.

While life-saving for many babies, ventilators carry more risks than CPAP and supplemental oxygen. Short-term complications include overstretching of the air sacs, which can lead to rupture and cause the lung to collapse (**pneumothorax**). Infection is also a big concern. The hosing contains water to keep the air humidified, but a warm, moist environment

Oliver and Victor needed breathing tubes and were on ventilators for the first 24 hours, then switched to CPAP. They managed well for the first few days but soon began to experience progressively more and more serious apneic spells. Soon they were struggling to keep their oxygen saturation above 80 percent, and I could hear the monitor alarm ringing in my head even when I stepped outside.

After 12 days on the CPAP, they each had breathing tubes inserted again and were back on a ventilator. There was no other option. It broke my heart, because they had struggled with all their might just to lift one foot from the starting line and now it felt as if we were taking 10 steps backwards. It was *day one* in the NICU all over again.

After the tears subsided, I realized I would only get through this one day at a time. I couldn't think about how things were last week, or what they would be like tomorrow, but only about what was happening right now. I circled a date on the calendar one week later and told myself I would think about it then. I called it my Scarlett O'Hara approach, and it has helped me through many dark times.

is the perfect place for bacteria and viruses to grow. In addition, the tube in the airways bypasses little hairs in the nose and mouth that normally trap bacteria (the lung's first line of defense against infection). The biggest long-term problem is **bronchopulmonary dysplasia (BPD),** a lung disease that interferes with oxygen transfer. The doctors will try to use the lowest safe level of breathing support to try to decrease the risk of BPD.

Therapies to Improve Lung Function

There are other important therapies to help improve lung function:

- **Maximizing nutrition.** Lung development and the process of healing lung damage uses a lot of calories. Some doctors also recommend additional vitamin A to reduce the severity of BPD.
- **Surfactant.** Artificial surfactant is administered down the breathing tube (endotracheal tube) into the lungs, where it coats the air sacs

(alveoli). Many babies receive surfactant in the delivery room during their initial resuscitation, and some will receive it later on in the NICU. Surfactant does not take care of all the issues caused by premature lungs, but it can improve lung function enough to allow lower pressure settings and oxygen concentrations. Sometimes a second dose is needed. Many babies less than 28 weeks receive surfactant and some between 28 and 34 weeks will also need it.

- **Bronchodilators** are drugs that open the airways, making it easier for oxygen to get to the air sacs. They can be inhaled (such as *albuterol, levalbuterol,* and *ipratropium*), administered by mouth (*theophylline*), or given intravenously (*aminophylline*).
- **Fluid restriction.** Fluid can accumulate in the space between the air sacs (alveoli) and the blood vessels, making it harder for oxygen and carbon dioxide to travel back and forth. Limiting intravenous fluids helps to keep the tissues dry, improving gas exchange.
- **Diuretics** are drugs that cause dehydration by eliminating more water through the kidneys. The first choice is usually *hydrochlorothiazide* and/or *spironolactone*. A stronger diuretic, such as *furosemide*, may also be used, but involves more side effects and may require monitoring of various blood levels.
- **Chest therapy** involves patting the back or applying vibration to loosen secretions.

How Long Will My Baby Need Oxygen?

As the lungs mature, the amount of respiratory support will be reduced; this is called weaning. The team will monitor how hard your baby is working to breathe, oxygen saturation, blood gas levels, and apneic spells. Depending on the individual factors, weaning off oxygen may take several days or could take many months.

For babies on a ventilator, weaning involves reducing the number of breaths supplied by the ventilator as well as decreasing the pressure and oxygen concentration. When a baby is breathing with minimal support from the ventilator, she will usually be transitioned to CPAP. As CPAP

On quiet nights one of the doctors would sit and talk with me to pass the time, a kindness I will never forget. When it became clear my boys would be going home on oxygen, I asked, "What will this lung damage mean?" His answer: "They will probably do just fine with everyday life, but will probably never climb Mount Everest."

I left the NICU about midnight, and on my way home I had to pull my car over to the side of the road because I was crying so hard. I had not cried for more than a month; we seemed to be making slow but steady progress, and I could finally see the light at the end of the tunnel. But here I was sitting in the dark, devastated over the idea that my boys would not be professional mountain climbers. If someone had phrased it differently and told me my boys would *want* to climb Mount Everest when they were older, my answer would have been a resounding "Over my dead body." The fatality rate is 30 percent, and I certainly wasn't spending all these nights worrying in the NICU to have them fall off a stupid mountain.

But there you have it: I was devastated. It made no sense, and yet it made all the sense in the world, because it was an acknowledgment of the loss of what might have been. When we look at our babies we think in terms of astronaut, president, and adventurer. A limitation, even a small one, is a crushing blow. Over the years I have adjusted to this. I wish I could tell you how, but I think it's just time; once you get your baby home the remnants of prematurity, including limitations, eventually start to fade into the background of everyday life. However, there is one thing I know for sure. No matter how well their lungs improve and how skilled they become, there is *no* way they are *ever* climbing Mount Everest!

offers less support, the oxygen concentration may be increased initially, to compensate. Think of this as a purposeful two steps forward and one step back.

A baby is weaned from CPAP by gradually reducing the pressure and the oxygen concentration. When minimal support is needed, trials with nasal prongs will be started, which means switching to supplemental oxygen via nasal prongs for a period of time and then back to the CPAP. Sometimes, alternating between CPAP and supplemental oxygen helps prevent fatigue because the extra support of CPAP allows some rest. Gradually, the amount of time spent on the CPAP round will be reduced.

Weaning off oxygen by nasal prongs involves gradually reducing the flow rate. When your baby is doing well on nasal prongs she may be started on room air trials, meaning removing the oxygen feed for progressively longer intervals to see if respiratory support can be stopped altogether. For weaning off an oxygen hood, the concentration of oxygen is gradually reduced to the level of room air.

When There Is a Problem Getting Off the Ventilator

Some babies have difficulty weaning off the ventilator. However, because a ventilator contributes to lung damage, the longer your baby needs this kind of the support the more difficult it becomes to transition to CPAP. Some options to help prevent further injury and get your baby off a ventilator include:

- **A high-frequency ventilator,** which delivers very shallow but rapid breaths. A regular ventilator is set to give less than 60 breaths per minute, but high-frequency ventilators allow hundreds of tiny breaths per minute. This breathing pattern may help minimize lung damage.
- **Nitric oxide,** which is a gas that dilates blood vessels, making it easier for oxygen to get from the air sacs into the blood vessels. It's mixed into the oxygen supply, but can have its own complications. It requires a very experienced team and is only indicated in particular circumstances.
- **An ultrasound to screen for pulmonary hypertension,** which is a narrowing of the arteries that carry blood from the right side of the heart to the lungs. This puts a strain on the heart, because it has to work harder to get blood through the narrow arteries. Treatment includes increasing the oxygen, nitric oxide, and the medication *sildenafil* (*Viagra*) to reverse the constriction.
- **Steroids** can be effective in helping a baby with damaged lungs transition from a ventilator but should be avoided in the first two

weeks of life as early use increases the risk of cerebral palsy and may also affect the way a baby's body and brain grow. Steroids also increase the risk of infection. While the infection risk is present no matter when steroids are given, the danger of affecting the nervous system lessens with time, so steroids may be given when a baby is three or four weeks old, when the risk of lung damage causing a handicap is greater than the risk involved in giving steroids.

7

The Cardiovascular System

The heart is a pump that provides the pressure to move blood to the lungs, where carbon dioxide is exchanged for oxygen, and also provides the pressure to pump this oxygen-rich blood from the lungs to the body. Just as the right water pressure is required to get water to all the taps in a house, the right blood pressure is required to get blood and oxygen to all the tissues. If the pressure is too low, oxygen delivery and waste removal will be suboptimal, and if it's too high, the pressure can damage the tissues and organs.

There is a network of sensors in the heart and throughout the body, providing constant feedback about oxygen levels, blood pressure, and a host of other factors, permitting an incredible degree of fine-tuning to match the body's ever-changing needs.

Cardiovascular Monitoring in the Intensive Care Nursery

The cardiovascular system is an important barometer of your baby's health, so every heartbeat is monitored. Three adhesive electrodes on the skin detect electrical activity in the heart, and the signal is translated into an image displayed in real time on a screen. The monitor can also detect irregularities in the heartbeat called **arrhythmias.** The tracing can be printed on paper for a closer evaluation if needed. Your baby's nurse is in charge of placing the electrodes and monitoring heart rate.

Blood pressure is actually two numbers: the **systolic pressure** (the pressure as the heart is contracting, or maximum pressure) and the **diastolic pressure** (the pressure in the system as the heart is relaxed and filling with blood). For a premature baby the normal systolic pressure ranges between 46 and 60 and the diastolic between 23 and 36.

Blood pressure is measured with a blood pressure cuff or with a catheter (like an intravenous device) in an artery, usually the umbilical artery or an artery in the wrist or foot. With a catheter, the pressure in the artery is translated into a waveform in an up-and-down pattern, just like an oxygen-saturation recording. The arterial catheter is more precise than a blood pressure cuff and gives a continual readout, which can be helpful when there are complex needs, but if your baby is not acutely ill, a traditional blood pressure cuff will be fine.

Other testing includes:

- **EKG (electrocardiogram),** a detailed recording of the heart's electrical activity. An EKG uses measurements from 12 electrodes, so it provides more information than the three electrodes used for monitoring heart rate. It's performed by a nurse or an EKG technician and is used to evaluate problems such as an irregular heartbeat (arrhythmia) or a murmur (a sound produced by abnormal blood flow in the heart).

- **Echocardiogram (echo),** an ultrasound of the heart that evaluates the structure and function. An ultrasound technician will perform the scan without moving your baby. Many babies less than 32 weeks will get an echo to screen for patent ductus arteriosus (PDA), a heart problem common among premature babies. Other indications for an echo include a heart murmur, persistent blood pressure problems, or difficulties weaning off the ventilator.

- **Central venous pressure,** a measurement of the blood pressure in the veins right before they enter the heart. This requires an umbilical vein catheter. The information it finds can be helpful in determining the cause of blood pressure problems.

The Cardiovascular System and Prematurity

Bradycardia

Bradycardia is a slow heart rate. When the heart is not pumping fast enough, the flow of blood to the lungs is reduced, oxygen delivery to the tissues suffers, and waste products accumulate. A slow heart rate can also lead to low blood pressure. For a premature baby, any heart rate less than 100 beats per minute is bradycardia, and below 60 beats per minute is dangerously slow.

Heart rate is controlled by the autonomic nervous system, the part of the nervous system that functions outside of our conscious control. There are two distinct divisions of the autonomic nervous system controlling opposing functions: the **sympathetic nervous system,** which increases the heart rate and the force of the heartbeat, and the **parasympathetic system,** which decreases the heart rate. These two parts of the nervous system typically work in an integrated fashion to control heart rate. For a premature baby, immaturity of these systems can lead to an abnormal slowing of the heart rate, so bradycardia is often a "normal" or expected part of prematurity.

Bradycardia can also be triggered by low oxygen levels, often due to apnea, or by stimulation such as eating or inserting a feeding tube.

My journal is filled with entries about bradycardias. My head would turn back and forth from monitor to monitor, and just as one boy recovered, the other would bottom out. Each time I was worried the next drop would be "the big one," and the nurses would be unsuccessful in their resuscitation attempts. I felt as if I were treading water, and with each bradycardia spell it was as if someone was giving me one more brick to hold. But looking at my journal, after several bad weeks the bradycardias lessened and gradually became less of a health concern.

I know how sick you feel when you see that monitor drop. Writing about my fears helped. So did talking with parents who were a few weeks ahead of us in the NICU. Seeing that someone else made it through was very helpful.

However, bradycardia may also be a warning sign of infection, bowel problems, a low blood count (anemia), or other medical problems. Therefore the medical team has to distinguish between "normal" bradycardia and bradycardia triggered by a medical problem that requires treatment. Clues that there may be more going on than a premature nervous system include spontaneous bradycardia episodes, the severity (how slow and for how long), and a trend toward more frequent and/or severe drops.

Treatment depends on the severity and any negative effects, such as changes in blood pressure or oxygen saturation. Options include:

- **Observation.** If the blood pressure and oxygen saturation are stable, the nurse will wait a few seconds (that feel like a lifetime) to see if your baby's own nervous system will kick in to increase the heart rate.
- **Stimulation.** This can be as simple as a light touch or more vigorous, such as firmly rubbing the back.
- **Increasing the respiratory support,** either more oxygen or more help with breathing.
- **Caffeine** if the bradycardia is due to apnea.

Hypotension

Low blood pressure, or hypotension, is very common, and the more premature, the greater the risk: 40 percent of babies between 27 and 29 weeks and more than 60 percent of babies between 24 and 26 weeks will have blood pressure problems. Low blood pressure affects the flow of blood and oxygen to the brain and other vital organs. Shock is a severe form of hypotension—a life-threatening drop in blood pressure that requires immediate treatment.

Like apnea and bradycardia, hypotension may be due to an immature nervous system (mostly a problem for babies less than 30 weeks), but it may also herald an underlying medical problem, such as:

- **Hypoxia** (low oxygen levels)
- **Bradycardia**

- **Anemia** (low blood count)
- **Dehydration**
- **Infection**
- **Heart problems**
- **Medication side effects**
- **Bleeding into brain**

The medical team will do a careful evaluation, check the vital signs (heart rate, oxygen levels, temperature), monitor urine output (low output suggests dehydration), and take specialized measurements from an umbilical vein catheter if one is in place. Lab tests, X-rays, and even an ultrasound of the head and/or the heart may be ordered.

Management of hypotension includes treating the underlying problem. Some babies will also need IV fluids to increase their blood pressure and some may need medications. The most commonly used drugs are *dopamine*, *dobutamine*, and *epinephrine*. Some babies need two of these drugs to maintain their blood pressure. Many babies under 30 weeks need these medications as part of their initial stabilization.

Patent Ductus Arteriosus

The right side of the heart pumps blood to the lungs, where the blood picks up oxygen. The oxygen-rich blood is delivered back to the left side of the heart, which pumps this blood to the body. A patent ductus arteriosus (PDA) is a structural problem that interferes with the circulation of blood between the heart and the lungs. (See Figure 6.)

During pregnancy, oxygen is supplied by the placenta, not the lungs, so the heart does not need to pump much blood to the lungs. The ductus arteriosus is a circulation shortcut that allows blood from the right side of the heart to bypass the lungs during pregnancy. The ductus arteriosus normally closes shortly after birth, allowing the lungs to take over from the placenta. Prematurity can affect this process, and the ductus arteriosus may not close. If the ductus arteriosus remains open, this is called a patent ductus arteriosus (PDA). With a PDA some of the oxygen-rich blood in the aorta meant for the body is diverted back to the lungs, which are now receiving too much blood. The extra blood in the lungs makes it harder to breathe. It can also cause apnea, low oxygen levels, blood pressure problems, and fluid in the lungs as well as put too much strain on the heart. This is called a **left-to-right shunt,** as blood from the left side of the heart is shunted back to the right side.

A PDA is related to gestational age and birth weight—the risk is approximately 50 percent among babies who weigh less than 1,750 g (3 lbs, 14 oz) at birth and is almost 80 percent among those who weigh less than 1,000 g (2 lbs, 3 oz). Because it's so common, every premature baby will be evaluated at birth. The most telling sign is a heart murmur; a sound produced by abnormal flow in the heart, but an echo (ultrasound of the heart) is required for diagnosis.

FIGURE 6: Patient Ductus Arteriosus (PDA)

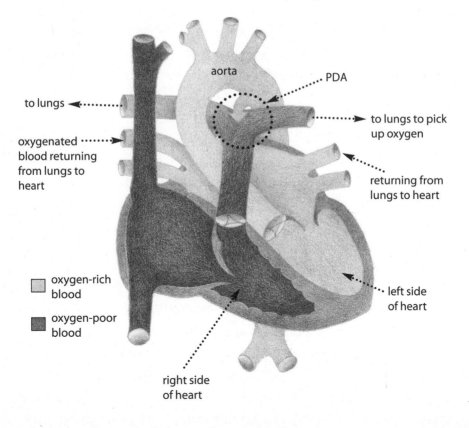

FIGURE 7: Algorithm for Managing a PDA

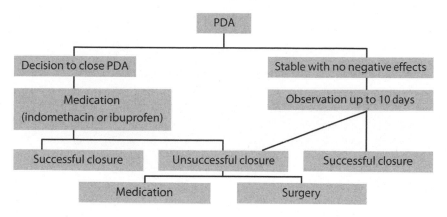

Treatment options for a PDA include:

- **Observation** for seven to 10 days if your baby is stable and the PDA is not contributing to apneas, bradycardias, or blood pressure problems. Approximately one-third of PDAs will close spontaneously; however, medication to close a PDA is less effective after this wait.

- **Medication,** either *indomethacin* or *ibuprofen,* will close 80 percent of PDAs. The risks of these medications include kidney and bowel problems as well as an increased danger of infection and bleeding. Babies with kidney problems, bleeding, infections, or **necrotizing enterocolitis** (a bowel condition, see chapter 12) may not be able to receive these medications.

- **Surgery** to tie the blood vessel shut. This is not open-heart surgery, because the heart is not opened. While it *is* scary, this is about as low-risk as heart surgery can be—the risk of death is less than 1 percent. The surgery may be performed in an operating room or even in the intensive care nursery on a radiant warmer, as the special ventilators for a premature baby are not found in most operating rooms and some babies may be too unstable to transport.

Regardless of where it happens, an experienced heart surgeon will perform the procedure, and an anesthetic will be given so your baby does not feel any pain.

"Why do you give *indomethacin* instead of *ibuprofen*?" I asked our neonatologist.

"That is what works best in our hands," he replied.

For me, as a doctor, that was the most satisfying answer possible. In situations where studies are not clearest on a single best option, like closing a PDA, the next step is the treatment that works best in *your* environment. Our neonatologist knew what worked with *his* people in *his* NICU.

So a doctor in Denver may recommend *indomethacin*, in Tampa the protocol may be *ibuprofen*, while the policy in Houston may be to wait and see if the vessel closes spontaneously. They may all be acceptable options. The important thing is that you *can* and *should* ask why—a good doctor will be happy to give you their best explanation.

Congenital Heart Disease

Congenital heart disease is a structural birth defect of the heart not related to prematurity. It affects 1 percent of children. There are many different defects, but the most common involve holes between chambers in the heart or structural abnormalities of the valves. Congenital heart disease strains the heart and lungs and, depending on the problem, may even cause damage. In some cases, the problem must be repaired almost immediately, other conditions can wait until your baby is older and bigger, and some do not require any treatment, as they typically improve as the heart grows.

There are too many unique defects with different therapies to discuss in this book; however, if your baby has a significant congenital heart defect *in addition* to prematurity, you should consult with a pediatric cardiologist (heart specialist).

Both Oliver and Victor received *indomethacin*. Victor's murmur resolved, but Oliver's did not. The assumption was that the *indomethacin* had been unsuccessful, but to be sure, another echo was performed. I listened in disbelief when I heard that Oliver had a large hole in his heart and a malformed valve that was affecting the flow of blood to his lungs. The hole could be observed, but the valve was another thing.

Surgery was needed, but he was too small: The only thing worse than hearing your baby needs heart surgery is hearing that he can't have it. He was still less than 800 g (1 lb, 12 oz) and needed to weigh 1,400 g (3 lbs, 1 oz) for the procedure. The paradox was that his heart problem made gaining weight more difficult.

Gram by gram, Oliver slowly gained weight. Six weeks later a tiny wire was threaded through a vein in his leg to his heart, and the valve was popped open. Where once the valve was too tight, now it didn't function at all. Still problematic, but less so. Sometimes there are no fixes, just a trade-off for a less serious problem. But I still consider us very lucky—a few years earlier the only solution would have been open-heart surgery.

8

The Nervous System and Prematurity

The nervous system is the most complex and intricate structure in the human body. It's one of the first organ systems to develop and the last to be completed. Therefore it's especially vulnerable to prematurity—even babies born at 35 or 36 weeks can have consequences. Complications affecting the nervous system, such as cerebral palsy, lower IQ scores, autism, and attention deficit disorder, are the most common disabilities for premature babies.

However, there are many interventions to help mitigate these effects. Understanding the nervous system, how it develops during pregnancy and after birth, and the effects of prematurity are the first vital steps in helping a premature baby reach her potential.

How the Nervous System Functions

The nervous system is an electric circuit that powers our every thought, action, and bodily function. It's also a sophisticated monitoring system that communicates real-time information about both the surroundings and the internal workings of the body.

The basic unit of the nervous system, the actual wiring, is a specialized cell called a **neuron.** Neurons are organized into three locations:

- **The brain** is both the command center and power plant for the nervous system. It is extremely complex, with one hundred billion neurons and more than ten thousand connections to and from the body. Only a small part of the brain is under conscious control; most of what happens occurs without thinking. The brain is divided into the **cerebrum** and the **cerebellum.** The cerebrum is divided into two halves, right and left, called hemispheres, which are organized primarily by function. As the nerve fibers leave the hemispheres, they cross over from one side to the other. This means that the nerves from the right side of the brain control the left side of the body and vice versa. The cerebellum is a relay center, which sits below the cerebrum. (See Figure 8.) It functions like an airtraffic controller, integrating vast amounts of sensory and motor information so every movement is precise. The brain receives nourishment from blood vessels and is bathed in a special fluid called **cerebrospinal fluid (CSF)** that flows around the brain and through channels in the brain called **ventricles.**

FIGURE 8: The Brain Showing Ventricles and Germinal Matrix

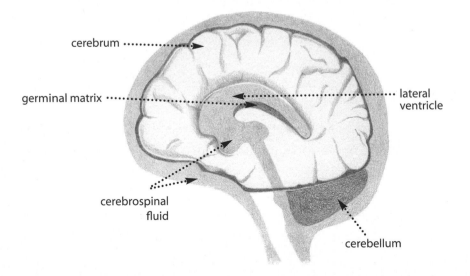

cerebrum

germinal matrix

lateral ventricle

cerebrospinal fluid

cerebellum

- **The spinal cord** relays messages back and forth from the brain to body. It's a superhighway, with a multitude of complex pathways. The spinal cord is also bathed in CSF.
- **The peripheral nerves** transmit and receive the electrical signals from the muscles, skin, and organs. Touch, smell, and sight—every feeling and physical sensation generates an electric current that travels along these nerves to the brain. Peripheral nerves also control muscles and movement. Some nerves are under conscious control (the ones that move our muscles), and others function under the control of the autonomic nervous system, which is like an autopilot keeping the heart beating, the lungs breathing, and the bowels moving.

The nervous system relies on complex signaling. Chemicals, hormones, and other substances called **neurotransmitters** are the flint, triggering an electrical signal in the nerve. For nerves to communicate, the electric signal must be translated back into a chemical message to pass from one nerve to another. Once it reaches the new nerve, the chemical message is then converted back into an electric signal. Think of it like a very intricate game of telephone. Some neurons are coated with **myelin,** a fatty substance that acts like insulating material. This allows the electric signal to move faster and keeps the electricity on the correct nerve.

In many ways the nervous system is like a computer. It comes with specific pre-installed hardware (such as control of the heartbeat or breathing), but new pathways can be created by experience and effort (such as eating or walking), just like loading software.

The nervous system is especially vulnerable to injury; damaged or destroyed neurons in the brain and spinal cord cannot re-grow if injured, although peripheral nerves can regenerate. While much of the nervous system cannot be replaced or even repaired, there's a safety mechanism called **neuroplasticity.** This is the ability of the nervous system to rewire itself in response to injury, so if one part of the system is damaged, often other neurons can compensate. This is like being in a railway yard. If a train track becomes damaged, the railroad switch operator throws a lever that guides the train to a functioning track. This is only possible in certain areas of the brain and with specific nerves; some areas have no ability to compensate for injury.

Prematurity and the Nervous System

Nervous system complications are generally related to one, or both, of these processes:

- **Injury** from bleeding, infection, or lack of oxygen. Inflammation, which is a response to injury, may be more damaging than the original insult.
- **Exposure of an immature nervous system to our hostile environment.** Before 37 weeks, a baby is designed to survive in the warm, dark, quiet, fluid-filled uterus. Because nervous system input is important in development, during pregnancy the nervous system amplifies signals that go to the developing brain. The main mechanism for this amplification process is a receptor called the **NMDA receptor,** which is found throughout the nervous system. It functions like a switchboard, receiving and amplifying input before sending it on to the brain. After birth, a change happens and the NMDA receptor starts muffling input. This helps us cope with the loud noises, bright lights, and other excessive input from the outside world. A premature baby may not be able to accomplish this switch for some time. This is like having a house where the wiring is not completely installed—if you start turning on the appliances too soon, you risk short-circuiting the system. This amplified input may affect development of the nervous system.

Neurological Evaluation

Every premature baby is closely evaluated for signs of neurological concerns. The physical signs that increase suspicion of a nervous system problem are:

- **Abnormal muscle tone.** Low tone, or **hypotonia** (muscles too weak), and high tone, or **hypertonicity** (muscles too tight), can be signs of a potential problem, although low tone is *normal* before 30 weeks gestation.
- **Asymmetry in posture or movement,** meaning that muscle tone or motion on one side of the body is markedly different than on the other.
- **Behavioral concerns,** such as lethargy, jitteriness, irritability, and feeding problems.
- **Abnormal vital signs** including problems with heart rate, breathing, blood pressure, and even temperature.
- **Seizure,** meaning uncontrolled twitching or shaking of the body.
- **Tense fontanelle.** The fontanelle is the soft spot in a baby's skull where the brain is only covered by membranes and the scalp. The fontanelle should be slightly depressed; if it is tense or full, this could mean too much pressure on the brain.
- **Abnormal reflexes.** A reflex is a muscle response out of our conscious control. Some reflexes are normal, others are primitive (normally present in babies but go away with time), and some are always abnormal.

Intraventricular Hemorrhage

Intraventricular hemorrhage, or IVH, is bleeding in or around ventricles of the brain (the channels that circulate cerebrospinal fluid). The bleeding happens in the first few days of life and occurs in a very important but fragile brain area called the **germinal matrix,** which is the floor of the lateral ventricle. The germinal matrix produces new nerve cells for the rapidly growing brain, so injury in this area can have significant consequences on brain growth and development.

Gestational age is the biggest risk factor for IVH, because the germinal matrix starts to shrink by 28 weeks and disappears by 35 weeks. Birth weight is also a factor: The risk of IVH is 20 percent for babies who weigh less than 1,500 g (3 lbs, 5 oz) at birth. Other contributing factors include blood pressure issues (too low or too high), problems with oxygen delivery during birth, and infection.

The amount of bleeding and the affected area of the brain are used to grade IVH.

- **Grade I,** bleeding into the germinal matrix only.
- **Grade II,** in which the bleeding has spread into the ventricles, but the ventricles are not distended.
- **Grade III,** meaning enough blood has accumulated in the ventricles that they have become distended and are compressing the surrounding brain tissue. This can cause reduced delivery of oxygen and nutrients as well as inflammation in the brain tissue, which is potentially damaging.
- **Grade IV,** wherein the blood has extended from the ventricle into the brain tissue and causes injury.

The risk of major nervous system complications increases with increasing grades of IVH. (See Table 1.) Grades III and IV hemorrhage are larger and are more likely to cause permanent injury to the developing brain. With a grade IV intraventricular hemorrhage it is important to factor in whether the bleeding has occurred on one or both sides of the brain (unilateral or bilateral). Approximately 4 percent of babies who weigh less than 1,500 g (3 lbs, 5 oz) develop a grade III or IV IVH.

All premature babies less than 32 weeks at birth and older babies with a birth weight less than 1,500 g (3 lbs, 5 oz) are at risk for IVH and will be screened with a brain ultrasound. The machines are portable, so the scan can be done in the NICU. The brain is scanned through the **fontanelle**—there is no bone in this area, so a clear image of the brain is possible. It's rare to miss an IVH with an ultrasound. A CT scan or an MRI is another option, but these scans require sedation and moving your baby out of the NICU, so they are only used when more detailed information is critical.

The first ultrasound is typically performed three to seven days after birth, although a scan on day one or day two may be indicated if there

TABLE 1: Risks Associated with Intraventricular Hemorrhage for a
Premature Baby Weighing Less than 1,500 g at Birth*

Grade	Moderate to severe cerebral palsy	Intellectual disability
No IVH	6%	11%
Grades I and II	13%	19%
Grade III	15%	30%
Grade IV unilateral	36%	36%
Grade IV bilateral	88%	93%

* These numbers are averages. Risks may be higher or lower based on individual factors.

are early signs of IVH, such as a drop in blood count or recurrent brady-cardia or apnea. Every baby with a grade II or higher requires a follow-up ultrasound about one week later, because they are at risk for **hydrocephalus,** a condition in which excess fluid accumulates in the ventricles, which can damage the brain. Ultrasounds will be performed on a regular basis until the blood has been reabsorbed; think of this as keeping an eye on a bruise until it disappears. The team will also closely monitor head circumference, as a rapidly enlarging head is a sign of hydrocephalus.

If hydrocephalus develops, the management options that could be discussed include:

- **Observation,** especially for mild hydrocephalus, which may resolve spontaneously in four weeks.
- *Acetazolamide,* a medication that slows production of cerebrospinal fluid.
- **A reservoir,** which is a thin catheter inserted in the ventricle that connects to a small bubble under the scalp. The procedure is performed by a pediatric **neurosurgeon.** Once the bubble is in place a needle can be inserted to withdraw fluid as needed.
- A ventriculoperitoneal (VP) shunt, a tube to drain fluid from the ventricles to the belly (the peritoneal cavity). This is also performed

by a neurosurgeon. A VP shunt cannot be placed until a baby weighs at least 2,000 g (4 lbs, 7 oz). Approximately 4 percent of babies with a grade II IVH, 18 percent with a grade III, and 29 percent with a grade IV will ultimately need a shunt.

Predicting the outcome for any baby with IVH is difficult, as the grade of the bleed only tells part of the story. Other factors that must be considered are your baby's gestational age, birth weight, infection, the size and location of the bleed, whether or not she develops hydrocephalus, and the need for a VP shunt. In addition, a condition called PVL (see below) will also affect prognosis. Some babies with IVH, even with severe bleeds, fare better than expected. This usually involves a monumental long-term effort from the family. For other babies, even with the very best of care in the hospital and at home, a grade III or IV bleed will mean serious medical issues, intellectual disability, and cerebral palsy.

Because so many babies with bilateral grade IV bleeds have very profound long-term health problems, after considering all of the individual

Waiting for that first ultrasound was like heading toward an unseen fork in the road. I could pray/hope/beg to have the easier path, but I had no control over the situation. Waiting for an ultrasound about your baby's brain *is* about the most worrying and stressful thing. Ever.

When the day finally arrived I must have checked in with the nurses every 15 minutes to see if the report was ready. Each time the answer was the same. "No, not yet."

That night our neonatologist came to my room with the ultrasound results. I was sure this personal visit meant the worst. "Their ultrasounds are fine," he said. "A grade II bleed, so it is unlikely to have a significant impact." He tried to reassure me by telling me that he himself could have had one at birth.

I suspected the last part wasn't entirely true, that no bleed was probably best; however, inside I was jumping for joy. It's a strange place to be, when you can be relieved your baby only had a grade II bleed. But there you have it.

variables and the amount of unaffected brain tissue, there are situations in which the option of withdrawing medical care may be discussed. Even though it's hard, ask to hear about both the best and the worst prognosis. Speaking with a pediatric **neurologist** may also be helpful. Understand that the information given is not a prediction, but information based on studies of premature babies who have experienced similar problems. This is a very difficult situation for parents, and different families will make different decisions based on beliefs, values, and other factors.

Periventricular Leukomalacia (PVL)

PVL is a brain injury caused by a lack of oxygen or blood flow to the brain that results in the loss of brain tissue around the ventricles. In severe cases there is so much loss of tissue that cysts develop in the brain—this is called **cystic PVL.** The periventricular area contains nerve fibers that carry messages from the brain to the muscles, so PVL is a serious injury that increases the risk of cerebral palsy, intellectual disability, and vision problems. (See Table 2.) PVL is not caused by intraventricular hemorrhage (IVH), but these two brain injuries may be seen together because they share the same risk factors: prematurity and low birth weight.

TABLE 2: Impact of PVL on Risk of Cerebral Palsy

Type of PVL	Risk of cerebral palsy
No PVL	5%
PVL without cysts	17%
Unilateral cystic PVL	35%
Bilateral cystic PVL	75%

A baby who weighs less than 1,500 g (3 lbs, 5 oz) is at greatest risk for PVL. The risk ranges from 4 percent to 26 percent depending on birth weight and a variety of other factors like gestational age, infection, needing a ventilator, and blood pressure problems.

Babies with PVL have no outward signs or symptoms, so every baby at risk will be screened with an ultrasound of the brain four to eight weeks after birth (evidence of PVL on ultrasound does not appear for several weeks). If the ultrasound suggests PVL, an MRI may be recommended to obtain more detailed information.

There is no treatment for PVL. What makes PVL and IVH so difficult is the fact that the long-term effects will not be known for many months. Some early signs of problems include persistent feeding difficulties and stiffness in the muscles.

Seizures

A seizure is an episode of abnormal and excessive electrical activity in the nervous system. When most people think of seizures, they think of the body shaking uncontrollably all over, but seizures with a premature baby are generally milder. The two most common types of seizures for a premature baby are:

- **Tonic seizure,** which affects muscle tone. The body repetitively stiffens up, either all over or just one part (like an arm or a leg).
- **Subtle seizure,** which involves repetitive subtle activities, such as eye blinking, staring, and mouth and tongue movements. Apnea can also be a sign of subtle seizure activity.

The most common causes of seizures are:

- **Brain injury due to low oxygen levels,** also called **hypoxic-ischemic encephalopathy.** This injury can occur before, during, or after birth.

- Intraventricular hemorrhage.
- Low blood sugar (glucose).
- Low blood calcium, magnesium, or sodium.
- Infection.

The management of seizures includes three essential steps:

- Ensure the oxygen level is adequate, and correct it if it's too low.
- Check blood levels of glucose, sodium, calcium, and magnesium, and correct them with IV medications if needed.
- Administer medications in the IV to stop the seizure. The most common ones are *phenobarbital, phenytoin,* and *lorazepam.*

It's also important to identify the cause of the seizure. Tests include:

- Checking for infection. Blood and urine will be tested and a spinal tap may be performed to check for infection around the brain. A chest X-ray to look for pneumonia may also be indicated. (See chapter 9 for more on infection.)
- EEG (electroencephalogram), a recording of the brain's electrical activity. It is painless and can help determine the cause of a seizure and the prognosis.
- An ultrasound to check for bleeding in the brain (IVH).
- MRI, which produces a detailed picture of the brain without the radiation of a CT scan. This will be performed once the seizures are controlled.
- CT scan, which also provides pictures of the brain. It's not as good as an MRI when it comes to evaluating seizures, so it's a second choice if MRI is not available.

The long-term effects of a seizure depend on the cause and the results from the EEG and MRI. It's important to sit down with the neonatologist and sometimes a neurologist to discuss the implications.

Developmental Care

Developmental care is based on the principle that environment makes a difference. The outside world is very stressful for a premature baby, and stress is physically damaging to a developing brain. Because a premature baby's nervous system is still wired to amplify input, even simple things like sound and touch can be very stressful.

Developmental care involves promoting the best environment for a developing premature nervous system. Health care professionals who work in the NICU can be specifically trained in these principles by an organization called the Newborn Individualized Developmental Program (NIDCAP). Premature babies who receive this kind of specialized developmental care in the NICU not only do better overall, but their brains show fewer physical effects of prematurity. This type of specialized care is a great way for you to make a difference.

According to NIDCAP, developmental care is centered on the following concepts:

- **"Organized" babies do better.** A nervous system that is coping well with the environment is *organized*; it's processing input and responding appropriately.
- **Changes in the environment can help a baby be organized.**
- **Subtle behaviors indicate stress and disorganization, or relaxation and readiness to interact with the environment.**
- **Family members are encouraged to be as involved as possible.** Learning subtle behaviors and cues will promote their baby's health and development.

Babies have ways of indicating their level of organization. Every baby is unique, so close observations help determine how an individual baby shows signs of stress. If a baby shows signs of stress, activities should be stopped (if possible) to allow the nervous system to rest and reorganize. Your baby's nurse will help you interact with your baby in the most positive manner. Some cues to watch for include:

- **Physiology** or how the body functions. The brain controls heart rate, respiratory rate, temperature, skin color, and movement, as well as gastrointestinal tract functioning. Signs of disorganized physiology include fast or slow heart rate or breathing, apneic spells, and dusky or blotchy skin color. Other signs of stress are startling, yawning, coughing, hiccoughing, sneezing, and spitting up.
- **Motor behaviors** such as muscle tone, posture (how a baby holds her muscles), and movement. An organized baby is flexed (arms and legs tucked in) with hands close to the face. Movements are fluid, with no twitching or tremors. A stressed baby may be stiff (hypertonic) or not have enough tone (hypotonic). Other stress signs are arching the back, lying with arms over the head, hands in a fist, and splayed fingers or toes.
- **Disorganized behavior,** which is a hyper-alert state (wide eyes, as though in a panic), looking away or staring, unpredictable episodes of crying, or agitation in response to touch or changes in environment.
- **Self-regulation,** which is the ability of a baby to organize the nervous system. Self-regulating behaviors include keeping hands to mouth or face, bringing hands or legs to the midline of the body, tucking arms and legs (swaddling), sucking, grasping, and looking.

Ways to promote a healthy nervous system in the NICU:

- **Limit interaction to organized times.**
- **Promote regular sleep cycles** with a blanket over the incubator to maintain a dark and quite environment.
- **Promote organized behavior** by swaddling to keep the arms and legs tucked, or gently bringing the hands to the midline or face.
- **Work with a specially trained occupational therapist.**
- **Provide a pacifier to suck.**
- **Skin-to-skin contact** with parents, also called **kangaroo care.**
- **Hold your baby during stressful procedures.**

One of the first things our nurse talked to us about was developmental care. She was very clear about how it could help and that we were key elements in the process. "Nurses will come and go on shifts," she explained. "You are the one constant factor." We were also given a booklet with pictures showing organized and disorganized behavior, and I studied it for hours. Our nurse was a master at tucking, and when the boys were agitated from a procedure, she had them swaddled up like a burrito and calmed down in minutes.

The more I learned about developmental care, the more I became a believer. It's one of the rare medical concepts that is simple, intuitive, and proven effective by research. Just knowing there were windows of opportunity to jump in and help my boys also took away some of that helpless NICU feeling. And so I sat with my boys as much as possible. I watched them and availed myself of every opportunity to swaddle them, hold them, and bring their hands to the midline. With every small activity I felt as if I were molding their nervous system just a little bit. And I think the healing went both ways.

9

Infection in the NICU

Premature babies are more susceptible to infections, and being hospitalized increases their risk of exposure. The consequences are significant. Infection can affect your baby's ability to breathe and to gain weight, and may prolong the hospital stay. Long-term consequences include an increased chance of chronic lung disease and cerebral palsy. Sadly, some babies will succumb to their infection. The good news is there are steps to take to prevent some of these infections, which in turn can have a profoundly positive effect on your baby.

What Causes an Infection?

Infections are caused by any one of three kinds of microorganisms:

- **Bacteria,** which are tiny, single cells found in the environment, on the skin, and in the gastrointestinal (GI) tract. Bacteria are treated with antibiotics.
- **Viruses,** which are organisms that are smaller than bacteria. They're not susceptible to antibiotics. Most viruses have no specific treatment, although a few can be treated with medications called antivirals.

- **Fungi,** also known as yeast. They are normally present in the GI tract and on the skin, but can cause potentially life-threatening bloodstream infections. Yeast infections are treated with antifungal medications.

A premature baby is more likely to catch an infection than a term baby because prematurity affects the body's developing defense mechanisms, including:

- **The skin,** which is the first line of defense. Intravenous needles and injections compromise this physical barrier. In addition, premature skin is so fragile that tape or excessive pressure can be damaging.
- **Immature lungs.** Microorganisms are more likely to get trapped in the smaller airways of a premature baby.
- **Bacterial imbalance.** The GI tract has a complex ecosystem of good bacteria, which aids with digestion, as well as potentially harmful bacteria. Prematurity, antibiotics, and lack of food by mouth can all upset this delicate balance.
- **Immature immune system.** It takes a few months after birth for the immune system to reach full development. A premature immune system is even more vulnerable and may be further weakened by medical and nutritional challenges.

Types of Infections

The five most common infections for a premature baby in the hospital are:

- **Skin infection,** typically at a site of skin breakdown or at an IV site. The infection may cause ulcers and can also spread to the bloodstream.
- **Pneumonia,** which is an infection of the lungs. It may be acquired during delivery or afterward in the hospital.

- **Urinary tract infection,** also known as a bladder infection. This type of infection is uncommon in the first few days.
- **Bloodstream infection,** which is the most common type of infection for a premature baby. Microorganisms may spread to the blood from another infection or from the GI tract, or they may be acquired before delivery via the umbilical cord.
- **Meningitis,** which is an infection of the fluid and membranes around the brain. It is typically a bacterial infection that has spread from the bloodstream.

Diagnosing an Infection

It's not easy to tell if a premature baby has an infection. Premature babies don't show typical signs such as fever or chills, and they can't tell us they are feeling unwell. Their communication tools include apnea, bradycardia, breathing effort, temperature, and changes in behavior such as tone, fussiness, or feeding difficulties. Unfortunately, these things are non-specific and can be the sign of any number of problems.

Tests to help diagnose an infection include the following:

- **White blood cell (WBC) count.** WBCs fight infection. A high or a low count is concerning. However, the test is not that accurate—only 10 percent of babies with an abnormal result actually have an infection.
- **Type of white blood cell.** Neutrophils are specialized WBCs that are produced by the body in response to inflammation and infection. During an infection, the body activates defenses very quickly, releasing immature neutrophils. (Think of this as mobilizing soldiers still in basic training.) The ratio of immature to total neutrophils may change in response to infection.
- **CRP level.** This stands for C-reactive protein, which is a substance released by the body in response to inflammation. An elevated result may indicate infection.
- **Chest X-ray.** This is the best test to identify pneumonia.

- **A nasal swab.** The inside of the nose is sampled for viruses that can cause pneumonia.
- **Spinal tap** involves removing a small amount of CSF (cerebrospinal fluid—the fluid that circulates around the brain and spinal cord) to test for meningitis.
- **A culture,** which involves trying to grow microorganisms to identify the exact type of infection. Almost anything can be submitted for culture including blood, urine, CSF, and even secretions. Culture results can also help guide antibiotic selection for a bacterial infection.

Because the risks associated with missing an infection are so high, the threshold for testing is very low. Many babies will be evaluated two or more times for infection during their stay in the NICU. It is frustrating, because some tests may be repeated over the course of several hours or days and false alarms are common. An early test, like a WBC or CRP, may suggest an infection, so treatment is often started while the other results are pending. Think of it this way: If your premature baby appears sick, she has to prove it's *not* because of an infection.

Pregnancy-related Infections

Infections within the first 72 hours are acquired before or during birth. The risk of a pregnancy-acquired infection is significant because 50 percent of premature babies are exposed to infection before or during delivery, although not all babies who are exposed will get sick.

Antibiotics will be started at birth if there is *any* concern about infection, because a delay of even a few hours while waiting for test results can affect the outcome. The most common regimen is a combination of two antibiotics, *ampicillin* and *gentamicin,* but antibiotic choices may vary from hospital to hospital. The specific microorganisms vary regionally, so your medical team will select the antibiotics that are most likely to be effective in your area of the country.

One of the first questions I asked was whether or not Oliver and Victor had infections. I was told they were on antibiotics.

"But what about their white cell counts?" Victor's was very low.

The next day I became sick. High fevers, shaking chills, and horrible sweats. I was getting the same treatment as my boys: blood tests, X-rays and scans, and IV antibiotics. Within 24 hours my blood cultures were positive for *E. coli*, a bacteria known for causing serious bloodstream infections. My particular strain was resistant to most antibiotics. All I could think was, "So this is what I've given my boys." It was like seeing *worst mother ever* in bright red letters on a marquee.

One of my OB/GYN colleagues sat me down and gave me a speech that I myself have given to hundreds of women: "You know this is not your fault. You did not do anything to catch this infection. If infection in pregnancy was easy to prevent, there would be two hundred thousand or so fewer premature babies every year in the United States."

I just needed to hear someone say it out loud.

Some test results will be available within an hour, but the full set of results will take 48 hours. Antibiotics are typically given by IV for 10 to 14 days if the tests indicate an infection. Decisions are more confusing if the results are negative. If every test is reassuring, the antibiotics may be stopped after 48 to 72 hours. However, if the risk of exposure to infection was very high (for example, you had a known infection before delivery or your membranes were ruptured for a long time) or some tests are abnormal (like the WBC count or CRP, but not the culture), antibiotics may be continued for four or five days, because the risks of an under-treated infection are very serious.

Hospital-acquired Infections

The risk of a baby catching an infection while in the NICU ranges from 6–33 percent. These hospital-acquired infections typically appear five or more days into the hospital stay. There are several sources of these germs:

- **Your baby's own bacteria.** Bacteria normally found on the skin can enter the bloodstream, typically in an area of skin breakdown or at an IV site. A premature baby can also develop leaky intestines, which allow bacteria from the GI tract to reach the bloodstream.
- **Equipment.** Bacteria, viruses, and fungi can grow on medical equipment, such as an IV catheter or in the tubing from a ventilator.
- **Caregivers,** both the medical team and family members, can unknowingly bring germs into the hospital and transmit them by touch, coughing, or sneezing.

Preventing hospital-acquired infections is essential. There are several ways to reduce your baby's risk. The first is focusing on clean hands. Touch allows microorganisms to leapfrog from person to person, or person to equipment. *Up to 60 percent of hospital-acquired infections are preventable with better hand hygiene.* Alcohol hand sanitizer is preferred: 20 seconds with sanitizer is better than 80 seconds with standard soap. Think of soap for visibly soiled hands (basically to remove dirt) and sanitizer for germs. Factors that increase germs on the hands include jewelry (sanitizer cannot get under rings and watches) and long-sleeved shirts. Alcohol sanitizer should be used before and after touching your baby. In addition, each baby should have a blood pressure cuff, stethoscope, and thermometer that is not shared with any other baby, as this equipment is not easy to clean between each use.

Insist that everyone use an alcohol sanitizer before and after touching your baby. Don't be afraid to speak up. It's okay to say, "I'm sure you just forgot, but could you please use the sanitizer?" In addition, if someone appears ill, he or she should not be caring for your baby. This includes you. If you're sick with a flu-like illness, stay home—you can pump milk and have someone deliver it for you.

Babies with an umbilical catheter or a **PICC (peripherally inserted central catheter, or PIC line),** a large IV in the arm or leg, are at increased risk for infection. These special IVs cause the majority of infections that develop after one week in the NICU. The longer the catheter is in place,

I worried every day about the PIC line. The specter of infection was a constant reminder of how all the ground we had struggled to gain could easily disappear. That is why I was so obsessed with getting the boys to tolerate their tube feeds, because the PIC line couldn't come out until they could eat.

On day 19 of their hospitalization, the boy's nurse greeted me with the biggest smile imaginable. The lines were coming out and the *nystatin* could be stopped. I was so excited that I cried. You would have thought they had graduated from Harvard!

the greater the risk of infection. PIC lines in particular increase the risk of yeast infection in the bloodstream, so as long as this kind of IV is in place, medication to prevent yeast infections may be given, either an IV medication called *fluconazole* or oral drops called *nystatin*. Meticulous attention to hand hygiene, a trained team for insertion and monitoring of the catheters, and replacing the catheter at 21 days also lowers the risk of infection. Using these techniques, some hospitals have gone more than two years without a single PIC line infection.

Medications may also play a role. Antibiotics kill bacteria; however, some bacteria survive and become more difficult to treat. (These are also called resistant bacteria.) Antibiotics can also contribute to the overgrowth of yeast. Other medications that increase the risk of infection are drugs for acid reflux and steroids.

When an Infection Is Severe

Sepsis is a severe whole-body response to infection. This can be the result of infection in the blood, but the infection can also be in the bladder (urinary tract infection), lungs (pneumonia), or bowel. Sepsis affects breathing, heart rate, and blood pressure and can damage the kidneys, heart, and brain. It may also affect the body's ability to form blood clots, leading to uncontrolled bleeding. (This is called **disseminated intravascular coagulation,** or DIC.)

Sepsis is a critical problem and requires skilled intensive care. Most babies with sepsis will need their own nurse. The treatment includes IV fluids, antibiotics, and help with breathing (usually a ventilator). Medications are often needed to help support blood pressure, and some babies will need blood transfusions. The medical team must also identify the source of the infection so it can be treated.

Vaccinations

Depending on the length of stay in the hospital, your baby may receive one or more vaccines before she leaves. Make sure the vaccines are given more than 72 hours before discharge so your baby can be observed for any side effects while she's still in the hospital. The last thing you want your first night home is an irritable baby with a mild fever.

Vaccination against hepatitis B, a viral infection that can cause liver damage and even liver cancer, is recommended at birth. The hepatitis B vaccine is less effective for babies who weigh less than 2,000 g (4 lbs, 7 oz), so for most premature babies it will be given shortly before discharge. There is one caveat: Hepatitis B can be transmitted from mother to baby during birth, so if you are hepatitis B positive, your baby should get the vaccine immediately at birth, regardless of weight.

If discharge is between late fall and early spring and your baby is eligible for RSV (respiratory syncytial virus) immunization, she should receive her first dose before leaving the hospital. See chapter 21 for more on the RSV and other vaccines.

Set aside half a day while your baby is in the hospital to review your own vaccination records and the records of anyone who will be in close contact with your baby. In particular, make sure you're up-to-date on the seasonal influenza and H1N1 vaccines (available every fall) and pertussis (whooping cough).

Blood: Understanding Tests and Disorders

B lood tests help manage nutritional needs, fine-tune respiratory support, and diagnose many medical conditions. In the first few days, some premature babies may need blood sampling as often as every one to two hours. Fewer tests are needed as the medical condition stabilizes. Most commonly, premature babies are tested for:

- **Complete blood count (CBC),** which is helpful in diagnosing infection, anemia (low blood count), and bleeding problems.
- **Electrolytes (sodium and potassium), calcium,** and **magnesium,** which are chemicals found in every cell and are an essential part of the body's internal communication system.
- **Glucose,** or blood sugar. Abnormalities are common due to complex nutritional needs and immature food processing systems in the liver and intestines.
- **Blood gas,** which indicates the levels of oxygen, carbon dioxide, and acid (pH) in the blood. (See chapter 6.)
- **Drug levels.** Some medications need close monitoring to ensure there is enough in the system to produce the desired effect. For other medications, testing is needed to make sure the level is not too high.
- **Bilirubin,** which is produced when red blood cells (RBCs) break down.

Out of all the procedures in the NICU, the heel sticks, though relatively innocuous, seemed the worst. It's hard to really understand what your baby is experiencing, but since I knew exactly how much a finger stick hurt, I could not only imagine how painful the procedure must be, but was also acutely aware that there was no way for my boys to process this kind of input.

It's hard to be a constant witness to pain, especially when it is your job to be calm, collected, and comforting. But I discovered even holding a finger or being close seemed to help them recover more quickly. I counted or softly sang to keep from getting worked up and looked away during the actual moment of pain; I still do. But being brave about smaller things, like heel sticks, also helped me to be brave about bigger things.

There are three methods for obtaining blood samples:

- **Heel stick.** Warm gel packs are wrapped around the heel to improve blood flow and then a sharp lancet is used to cut the skin.
- **Umbilical catheter** or **PIC line,** if present. This is painless.
- **Venipuncture.** A needle is inserted into an arm, leg, or scalp vein to withdraw blood.

Repeated painful procedures, such as heel sticks, are stressful for babies. The nursing staff will perform pain assessments during procedures (and at other times as well) and alert your baby's providers when more pain control is needed. Options for pain control include:

- Pacifier with sugar.
- Tight swaddling in a blanket.
- Cuddling with a parent during the procedure.
- Pain medications.

Jaundice

Jaundice is a yellowing of the skin due to accumulation of bilirubin in the blood. Bilirubin is a by-product of the body's recycling of red blood cells. High levels occur when the premature liver is overwhelmed and cannot remove bilirubin fast enough. (During pregnancy it's cleared by the placenta.) This becomes a problem because high levels of bilirubin are toxic to the nervous system. In addition to an immature liver, other causes of high bilirubin in a premature baby include:

- **Shorter life span of premature RBCs.** More frequent recycling produces more bilirubin.
- **Bruising.** A fragile premature baby is easily bruised during delivery. Bilirubin is released as the bruise is reabsorbed. (Bilirubin is what turns a bruise yellow.)
- **Medical concerns** such as dehydration, infection, and other health problems that affect the processing of bilirubin.

A premature nervous system is more vulnerable to the toxic effects of bilirubin, so every premature baby will have a bilirubin level (total serum bilirubin, or TSB) checked within 24 hours of birth and monitored closely to make sure it is not rising. If the bilirubin level rises above a certain level, based on birth weight and/or gestational age and the presence of other medical conditions, therapy is indicated.

Additional blood tests may be performed to look for other causes of elevated bilirubin. The most common cause is **isoimmunization,** a condition in which the mother produces antibodies that cross the placenta and attack the baby's RBCs when their blood types are incompatible.

The most common treatment for high bilirubin levels is light or phototherapy. Light, especially in the blue-green wavelength, converts bilirubin to less-toxic products easily removed by a premature liver. Babies who are smaller or facing more medical challenges will receive treatment at a lower bilirubin level because they are more susceptible to the toxic effects of bilirubin.

Phototherapy is accomplished by one of two means: special overhead lamps (often called **bili lights**) or a blanket with fiber optic lights (a **bili blanket**) on which a baby lies. Maximizing skin exposure to the light is essential, so only a diaper is worn and no swaddling is allowed. For many premature babies with low birth weight and other medical complexities, aggressive phototherapy is needed, so both methods are used.

Protective eyewear, even if the eyelids are fused, is necessary at all times to protect your baby's retinas. Temperature must be closely monitored to prevent overheating, as the lamps and blanket are both a heat source.

Some babies may need several days of phototherapy. The bilirubin levels are closely monitored to ensure they are dropping. When the TSB has been reduced to a safe level, phototherapy will be discontinued; however, the levels will be checked for a day or two afterward in case they rise again and a second course of phototherapy is required.

Phototherapy is sometimes not enough to control high bilirubin. In this case, a special kind of blood transfusion called an **exchange transfusion** is needed. This involves removing blood (and therefore bilirubin) and replacing it with a blood transfusion. It is a very fast way to get potentially dangerous levels under control. A very delicate procedure, the transfusion requires precise calculations, close monitoring, and experienced personnel. Fortunately, fewer and fewer premature babies are requiring exchange transfusions because of the availability of aggressive phototherapy.

Anemia

Anemia is also called a low blood count, meaning that fewer red blood cells (RBCs) are in circulation. RBCs carry oxygen, so anemia can contribute to hypoxia (low oxygen levels) and affect the ability to grow and cope with illnesses such as infection.

All babies, term and premature, develop a mild anemia in their first two to three months. The oxygen a baby receives during pregnancy is much lower than what we get from the air we breathe. To cope during pregnancy, babies have a special kind of hemoglobin, the oxygen-carrying molecule, which is more efficient at collecting oxygen and delivering it to the tissues. With the first breath, a baby is exposed to oxygen levels that are much higher than those in the uterus. This blast of oxygen temporarily halts production of RBCs in the bone marrow. As the old cells are removed from circulation, the blood count gradually drifts lower and lower. This situation corrects itself by two to three months of life when RBC production starts up again and a balance between RBC destruction and production is achieved.

In addition to this expected anemia, there are other reasons a premature baby develops a low blood count:

- **Excessive blood loss** from blood tests, bruising from delivery, and IVH (intraventricular hemorrhage). Blood testing is the *single most important factor* in anemia for a premature baby.
- **Shorter RBC life span** in a premature baby means the RBCs are removed faster from circulation.
- **Decreased RBC production.** Premature bone marrow is not ready to meet the demand for RBCs. Nutritional deficiencies, especially iron (a key component of hemoglobin), compound this problem.

The key to limiting the extent of anemia is a very conservative approach to blood samples. *Every* blood draw must have a reason, and you should feel empowered to ask, "How will the results of this test change my baby's health?" If there isn't a good answer, the test may not be needed. Adequate nutrition is also essential in preventing anemia.

Prevention of anemia may also include a medication called *erythropoietin* that stimulates the bone marrow to increase RBC production. *Erythropoietin* is an injection, and although the effect is not immediate, it can be very helpful in preventing the blood count from drifting downward over the first two to three months.

Some babies will need a blood transfusion. When deciding about transfusions, the medical team will look at your baby's hematocrit, which is the percentage of blood volume made up of red blood cells. However, the guiding principle with blood transfusions is not the actual blood

Oliver was severely bruised from head to toe at birth. Within a few hours after his delivery, a nurse practitioner arrived asking for permission for a blood transfusion. Oliver needed one now and Victor would in a few days, so we signed consents for both boys.

My heart skipped a beat. I had consented thousands of people for blood transfusions over my own career with similarly reassuring words: The risk of catching HIV from a transfusion is 1 in 1.8 million, yet here I was worried about that very complication. Clearly his immediate health concerns far outweighed almost one in two million, but I still couldn't shake the negative feelings.

I decided to tour the blood bank. As a physician, I had spoken with the technicians numerous times, but had never visited before. After meeting the technicians and learning about the screening process, I saw how fiercely protective they were about their tiny charges, whom they had never even met. They knew they were making a difference, and I was humbled by their dedication and professionalism.

I spent a lot of time wondering why I was so worried. It wasn't logical, but feelings never are. Having just come through an unusual pregnancy, losing one son, and with two others critically ill, I felt like a lightening rod for bad medical outcomes. I bet many parents of preemies feel the same way. Fears, realistic and otherwise, are normal. Acknowledging my fears, accepting that they were a normal response, and gathering more information helped me to move on.

count, but *how well an individual baby is coping with that blood count*. While each nursery will have a policy, a common approach is to use blood transfusions to keep the hematocrit at about 30 percent for a baby who is ill or on a ventilator. In convalescent premature babies, blood transfusions will be used to keep the hematocrit above 25 percent, and blood transfusions are recommended at a hematocrit of 18 to 20 percent even if there are no signs of anemia.

Most blood banks that serve NICUs have special donor programs and use a pool of very low-risk blood donors for premature babies. This is not only to reduce the risk of infections like HIV, but also because premature babies need to receive blood that is free of a virus called **CMV**

(cytomegalovirus). About 30 percent of people carry this virus. It might produce symptoms similar to influenza or mononucleosis (mono), but nothing serious for a healthy immune system. However, a premature baby can be seriously affected or even die from CMV. Special treatment can also be used to remove CMV from the blood. Blood is also screened for hepatitis B and hepatitis C as well as West Nile Virus and syphilis.

A premature baby will not use an entire unit of blood for a transfusion. Any blood not used can be kept up to six weeks for additional transfusions. This lowers the risk of transfusion-related infections by limiting the number of individual donors. For example, a baby who needs three blood transfusions over six weeks can receive all the blood from the same unit. It's not uncommon to check a blood count the day before a unit of blood is due to expire and give a transfusion even if the blood count is not that low, in the hopes that topping off the level will reduce the need for a later transfusion from a second unit of blood. Friends and relatives who have matching blood types can also donate blood. This is called a

My secretary, Gail, always brought a smile, gossip, and practical advice she was not shy about sharing. She also made sure the right news got through to the right people. She was the first person to visit after the boys were born, arriving right after we signed the consent for Oliver's transfusion. Although I don't remember, I must have told her about the transfusions and both of the boy's blood types, because within the hour one of the other administrators, Jane, was in my room announcing she was a low-risk, regular donor and was ready to give blood for Victor as they were both A-negative. And then off she went to the blood bank.

I was touched by her gift. It made me feel as if I had a secret army watching my boys, and when General Gail reported the latest development to the troops, a volunteer was happy to step forward, even before the question was asked. This is when I really understood that most people want to help and to comfort, even acquaintances that we might not know so well. Everyone I knew felt our suffering and wanted to make it just a little bit better. And help can come in many ways—a smile, words of encouragement, or even a unit of blood.

directed donation. The blood from a directed donation will not be ready to use for several days to allow for processing as well as screening for infections. Subsequent donations by the same person may be available for use sooner.

Disseminated Intravascular Coagulation (DIC)

In this disorder the blood loses the ability to clot. For a premature baby, infection and necrotizing enterocolitis (see chapter 12) are the most common causes, but other illnesses can trigger this condition. DIC is very serious. Without the ability to clot, bleeding can occur spontaneously in any area of the body (such as the brain or the abdomen), leading to many complications and even death. Treatment involves identifying the underlying cause, because it is essential to correct the triggering event. The other part of the care includes replacing clotting factors with specialized transfusions and correcting the anemia due to the blood loss.

Screening Blood Tests

All babies, regardless of gestational age, receive at least three tests at birth to screen for potentially serious conditions. There are about two dozen screening tests offered in the United States, but individual states regulate newborn screening, so the actual testing varies considerably from state to state.

Screening for hypothyroidism (low levels of thyroid hormone) is one of the three tests required in every state. The thyroid hormone controls metabolism, functioning of many organ systems, growth, and development. It's produced by the thyroid gland, which is found in the neck. Identifying a thyroid deficiency at birth is essential, as low levels can cause irreversible damage to the nervous system, such as lowering the IQ and increasing the risk of cerebral palsy.

Low thyroid levels are common among preterm infants. For some babies this is a temporary issue, related either to an immaturity of the thyroid gland or even a response to being sick. Some researchers believe a low thyroid level, which reduces the body's energy needs, might actually be a protective mechanism allowing a premature baby to survive with fewer energy requirements. An abnormal thyroid level may also represent a medical condition that would have existed regardless of prematurity.

The newborn screening test checks a thyroid hormone called T4, the most important hormone in diagnosing hypothyroidism. If the result is abnormal, more testing is needed, such as:

- **Free T4 assessment.** This tells how much of the actual thyroid hormone is available for the body to use.
- **TSH test,** which measures levels of the hormone that stimulates the thyroid gland. An elevated TSH indicates the body is trying to stimulate production of thyroid hormones.

Replacement of thyroid hormone is necessary if blood tests indicate hypothyroidism. Levels will be checked every few weeks after therapy is started to make sure the free T4 rises to the normal range and the TSH decreases to less than 10. The replacement usually comes in tablet form.

Victor had an abnormal thyroid screen, and of course his free T4 and TSH were abnormal. I tried not to be paranoid, but the risk of a thyroid disorder at birth is about one in four thousand.

There are times I wonder how much of Victor's cerebral palsy is thyroid related, and then I stop myself, because it doesn't really matter. Yes, premature babies with low thyroid function have a higher incidence of CP, but in Victor's case it was corrected, and whatever the cause of his CP, he had the right therapy.

I have come to realize that outcome depends on perspective. It's unfortunate to have a thyroid disorder, but it's fortunate to be diagnosed shortly after birth when corrective action can be taken. There were plenty of opportunities for worse outcomes.

A tablet is better than the liquid, as the medicine does not distribute evenly in the bottle, and so the doses can be inaccurate. Thyroid replacement should only be given with water. Iron in formula or breast milk can inactivate the medication, as can soy. While a feeding tube is in place, the tablet is crushed and flushed down the tube into the stomach. Once the feeding tube is gone, the tablet is crushed, mixed with a small amount of water, and squirted into the mouth against the inside of the cheek. Any time the dose or method of delivery is changed, the thyroid levels should be checked two weeks later.

~~~~~~~~~~

11

Nutrition and Feeding
in the Hospital

Premature babies need more energy to meet their everyday needs, such as breathing and staying warm. In addition, they must catch up on growth missed during pregnancy and often face physically draining medical challenges, such as infection and lung damage.

Feeding within the first 24 hours improves outcomes. While in the hospital, most premature babies will need between 110 and 140 calories per kg of body weight every day—this is 10 percent to 40 percent more than a term baby. The combination of protein, fat, carbohydrates, vitamins, and minerals they require is also different.

Your baby's growth will be monitored closely to ensure she is receiving adequate nutrition. Measurements will be plotted on a growth curve and include:

- **Weight.** A weight loss of 10 to 15 percent is expected in the first week and then the aim is a weight gain of approximately 1.5 percent of body weight every day (for example, a weight gain of 15 g a day is the goal for a baby weighing 1,000 g); however, this is usually two steps forward and one step back.
- **Length and head circumference,** which is measured weekly.

It was devastating to see Oliver and Victor lose weight. The scale dipped lower and lower, until Victor had dwindled to 777 g (1 lb, 11 oz) and Oliver to 655 g (1 lb, 7 oz). It was as if they were disappearing before my eyes.

I was in the waiting room worrying when another mother joined me. She did not speak English, but with my rudimentary medical Spanish I was able to understand that her daughter had also been born extremely premature and had been in the NICU for many weeks, but was almost ready to go home.

It was all too much. I managed to explain that my boys were losing weight, and then I started to cry. I wanted to tell her about my fears, but my Spanish failed me and I just couldn't find the words. It didn't matter, because she knew. She hugged me tight and we sat there for the longest time as she held me and comforted me.

The next day her daughter was discharged home. She came to find me, showed off her beautiful daughter, and gave me the biggest smile and a hug. I will never forget her face or how much she helped me just by understanding my fears. In the darkest of times, the most comfort comes from someone who has been there.

Intravenous Nutrition

Many premature babies will be fed initially via an IV, because their immature gastrointestinal tract may not be able to handle food. Babies who weigh less than 1,500 g (3 lbs, 5 oz) and those with complex medical needs and/or blood pressure problems are most likely to need intravenous nutrition.

There are two options: **peripheral nutrition,** which provides some nutrition, and **central nutrition,** which meets all nutritional needs. The choice depends on several factors, including the degree of prematurity, birth weight, medical concerns, nutritional needs, and when full tube feeds are expected to start. (See Table 1.)

When we eat, nutrients are absorbed from the bowel and sent to the liver, which acts like a Fed-Ex hub, processing and repackaging nutrients for delivery to the body and removing potentially harmful substances for disposal. Administering nutrition in the IV bypasses the liver and all of

TABLE 1: Peripheral Nutrition (PN) versus Central Nutrition (CN)

	Advantage	Disadvantage	Most appropriate for
Peripheral nutrition	Can use regular IV Lower risk of infection	Does not meet all nutritional needs, as regular IV is small and limits concentration IV lasts a few days, so frequent replacement necessary	Augmenting nutrition for a baby taking some tube feeds Full tube feeds expected within one week
Central nutrition	Meets all nutritional needs	Greater risk of infection from large IV (PIC line)	Full feeds not expected within one week

its checks and balances, so close monitoring is essential. An important team member in the NICU is the nutritionist, who will follow your baby's growth and development and make changes in the nutrient mix according to your baby's individual needs.

Monitoring will include weighing your baby daily and also weighing diapers to track fluid output. Many blood tests are needed in the first few days, but eventually only the blood sugar (glucose) will be tested daily, and other lab assessments, such as liver and kidney tests, will be performed once or twice a week (although protocols may vary). Every effort is made to limit these tests to prevent anemia (low blood count).

The most concerning risk is infection, especially with central nutrition—the high sugar and fat content of the solutions is a good place for bacteria to grow. (See chapter 9.) Gallbladder problems may also occur, especially for babies who need prolonged central nutrition and weigh less than 1,000 g (2 lbs, 3 oz).

Tube Feeding

Tube feeds are started when the gastrointestinal tract can handle food but a baby is not yet ready to try nursing or using a bottle. A tube from the nose (nasogastric, or NG, tube) or mouth (orogastric, or OG, tube) delivers breast milk or formula to the stomach. With feeding tubes, a baby doesn't need to have achieved the neurological maturity necessary to co-ordinate the mechanics of eating and breathing, and the tubes also elim-inate the energy expenditure of eating. Babies less than 32 to 34 weeks and older babies who are too sick to eat will be tube-fed initially.

Before 32 weeks, an OG tube is typically used, as the nose is so tiny that an NG tube can interfere with breathing. Babies needing nasal CPAP (see chapter 6) will also need an OG tube. When your baby is ready to try eating, the OG tube will be switched to an NG tube, because a tube in the mouth can physically interfere with eating.

Feeds may be given in several ways. How they are started and ad-vanced depends on gestational age, weight, and any medical conditions. Feeding options include:

- **Trophic feed,** which is a slow rate of infusion (sometimes called trickle feeds). Protocols for trophic feeds vary significantly. They do not provide enough calories to meet your baby's nutritional needs, but promote healthy bowels. Most babies under 32 weeks are started with trophic feeds.
- **Continuous feed.** With this type, the nutritional requirements for the day are calculated and the food is given continuously over 24 hours.
- **Bolus feed,** which is a meal every two to three hours.

Close observation is required to make sure your baby is tolerating tube feeds. Concerning signs are bloating (increase in abdominal girth) and excessive food that has not emptied from the stomach to the bowels, which is called a **feeding residual.** The stomach contents are withdrawn via the NG or OG tube before the next meal to check the feeding residual.

A high residual is 33 to 50 percent of the feed volume for bolus feeds, or more than one hour's worth of continuous feeds. Bile in the residual also indicates a baby is not tolerating tube feeds.

Feeding intolerance is more common among babies who weigh less than 1,000 g (2 lbs, 3 oz). The first treatment is to decrease the infusion rate, but some babies even have problems handling trophic feeds. Other options include:

- **A transpyloric tube,** which is a feeding tube that passes through the stomach and ends in the duodenum (the first part of the small bowel). A transpyloric tube will help if the problem is a sluggish stomach. Residuals must *not* be checked with a transpyloric tube, as the lining of the bowel can be damaged.
- **Changing feeds** for formula-fed babies so the food is not as rich and is easier to digest. Options may include changing to a formula with fewer calories or switching to predigested formula, which is easier for the bowel to handle. Predigested formulas include *Pregstamil, Alimentum, Nutramigen, Neocate,* and *EleCare.* Donor breast milk, if available, is an even better option.

Feeding By Mouth

Babies born between 32 and 34 weeks who are medically stable may try breast- or bottle-feeding. Babies who have been tube fed will be allowed to try eating when they are 32 to 34 weeks adjusted age. Several milestones must be met to eat safely:

- **Ability to coordinate sucking and swallowing,** which is not generally present until 32 to 34 weeks gestational or adjusted age.
- **Breathing without the help of machines,** although oxygen by nasal prongs is fine.
- **Respiratory rate less than 60 breaths per minute,** as faster breathing makes it difficult to coordinate eating and breathing, increasing the risk of food ending up in the lungs instead of the

stomach. Some babies with a respiratory rate up to 70 breaths per minute may be able to eat if they do not appear to be working hard at breathing.

- **Intestinal tract must be sufficiently mature** to digest and absorb food. This is rare for a baby less than 28 weeks. A buildup of stomach secretions or bloating indicates that the intestines are not ready for food.
- **Medically stability,** because apnea, bradycardia, and problems with blood pressure can affect sucking and swallowing. In addition, your baby should be alert enough to eat.

Many premature babies have difficulty learning to eat. Babies who are tube-fed for three or more weeks are at greatest risk. Some babies may develop an oral aversion, a condition where food or any oral stimulation is disturbing. Signs of oral aversion are crying, gagging, turning the head, or other avoidance tactics when food is offered.

Learning to eat is a matter of persistence, repetition, and developing endurance. An experienced NICU nurse, a lactation consultant, and an occupational therapist can all provide help. It's important to be prepared for slow progress. For example, 1 to 2 ml (less than a teaspoon) is considered a success with the first few attempts. Some babies are unable to master eating before discharge and will go home with a feeding tube.

Depending on your baby's nutritional needs, you may be able to try breast-feeding or may need to give pumped milk or formula in a bottle. Most bottle-fed babies are started with a soft, low-flow nipple that prevents them from getting too much milk in the mouth at once; however, it's not unusual to try several different nipples before settling on the right one. If the milk flows too fast, your baby might gag or choke. If the rate is too slow, your baby will use too much energy to feed. Babies suffering with gas due to air swallowed at feeding may be switched to an angled bottle, or nursing bags may be added. A pacifier can help in the transition from tube feeds to breast or bottle. This will not cause nipple confusion, but rather helps strengthen the muscles and develop the sucking reflexes.

Each hospital will have its own protocol, but in general the breast or a bottle is initially attempted once a day, because eating uses calories and can tire your baby. If your baby has not finished eating in 20 to 30 minutes, the remainder of the feed will be administered via the feeding tube. If you are breast-feeding, your baby will be weighed before and after each feed to gauge her intake. (One g of weight gain equals 1 ml of breast milk.) Additional attempts by mouth are added when a full feed can be completed in 20 to 30 minutes without signs of exhaustion, gagging, choking, apnea, or bradycardia. The feeding tube will be left in until full feeds are well tolerated for a day or so.

Breast-feeding and Milk Supply

Breast milk is the easiest food to digest and has antibodies that provide a much-needed boost to your baby's immune system. Breast milk is also one of the most important factors in protecting your baby from necrotizing enterocolitis, a very serious bowel problem. (See chapter 12.).

Breast milk may not have enough calories, protein, and calcium for a premature baby; at term, breast milk has 20 calories per 30 ml (1 oz), and many premature babies need 22 to 30 calories per 30 ml, depending on their birth weight and medical challenges. The calories in breast milk increase for about four weeks after a premature delivery, so breast milk alone is often adequate for a premature baby who weighs more than 1,500 g (3 lbs, 5 oz) at birth. Human milk fortifier, a powder that increases calories and other nutrients, can be added to breast milk for babies less than 1,500 g and those with greater nutritional needs.

Establishing your milk supply early is important. Most mothers have to pump. Many babies are too premature or too sick to start eating their first day, and you may be physically unable to get to the NICU. Even if you are able to breast-feed, the NICU still needs to have milk on hand, because you may not be able to be there 24 hours a day, and some premature babies tire out when they first start eating and may need some of their feeds supplemented via a tube. Your milk will be stored in a freezer in the intensive care nursery. Labeled containers will be provided so there is no chance of a mix-up.

It's important to start pumping as soon as possible after delivery and to try to pump eight times in 24 hours. This will help your milk to come in. During the first few days your body makes **colostrum.** Even though there will not be much initially, every drop is important, because colostrum is especially rich in infection-fighting antibodies. If you're able to breast-feed your baby, go to the NICU for as many feeds as possible, as this is the best way to establish your milk supply.

Problems with milk supply are unfortunately common. Pumping is a less efficient stimulus, and physical illness and stress also play a role. Be proactive and ask to meet with a lactation consultant, even if you appear to have a lot of milk. There's a lot to learn, and lactation consultants have much to offer. They will design the right regimen for you.

Suggestions for improving your milk supply include:

- **Use a commercial-grade electric pump.** These are rented, often by the hospital.
- **Pump both breasts at the same time.**
- **Pump for 15 minutes every two hours to get your supply started.** Once your milk supply is established, you can pump every three to four hours. The more you pump, the more milk you will have.
- **Metoclopramide (Reglan),** a medication that increases milk production. It will be prescribed by your OB/GYN. Metoclopramide may take a week or more to start working.
- **Fenugreek and blessed thistle.** These are herbs that increase production of breast milk. The dose for fenugreek is 1,200 to 2,400 mg three times a day. Many breast-feeding experts recommend slowly increasing the dose until your sweat and urine smell like maple syrup. The dose of blessed thistle is 700 to 1,450 mg three times a day. Fenugreek and blessed thistle often work best if you take both. They also work quickly, so if you have not seen an improvement in milk supply within a week, they will probably not work for you. Always discuss any herbs you plan to take with the lactation consultant and the neonatologist.

Knowing the benefits of breast milk, I was desperate to provide milk. But my supply was low, even with the strongest pump, regular pumping, and metoclopramide. I didn't realize how low until I noticed what the *other* mothers were leaving in the NICU freezer—veritable milk jugs compared to my little bags with 20 cc (1½ tablespoons). So I drilled the lactation consultants, redoubled my efforts, and took herbs, but I only succeeded in driving myself crazy. At my peak, five weeks after the boys were born, I managed 150 ml (5 ounces) total on a good day. In the beginning this was sufficient, as my boys were tiny and needed little. However, as they grew, my body, too sick, weak, and stressed, could not keep up. By six weeks their feeds were three-quarters formula and one-quarter breast milk.

I wasn't sure how much more of the pumping, with next to nothing to show for it, I could take. I already felt guilty about delivering prematurely, and now the posters aimed at promoting breast-feeding seemed to jeer, "What a bad mother you are."

Eventually, I spoke with one of the neonatologists. I told her how even the lactation consultant had suggested I quit (and in all my years as an OB/GYN I had never heard that). She smiled and nodded as she listened to my fears and concerns.

"Yes, breast milk is best," she said. "But it isn't always an option. Many moms with premature babies just can't make enough milk." And before I could reply she asked, "Were you breast-fed?"

I was caught off guard. "No, no I wasn't," I replied.

"You were probably fed some god-awful mixture of cow's milk and corn syrup," she added. "A pretty poor formula."

She was right.

"Well," she continued, "you turned out okay." And then she added, "You gave them five weeks of breast milk, and it has done them the world of good. Don't undo it all by driving yourself crazy. Remember, you can only do what you can do."

I stopped pumping that night.

I thought a lot about those words. They have become my second mantra, and when I am overwhelmed I say them out loud. I can only do what I can do, and I just have to let the rest go.

Donor milk, supplied by a milk bank, is another excellent option if breast milk is unavailable. A breast milk bank operates like a blood bank. Donated milk is screened for infections, such as HIV, and the milk is pasteurized to ensure it's free of bacteria and viruses. The pasteurization process does destroy some of the benefits. The protein and mineral content of donor milk is not sufficient to promote growth and development over the long term for a premature baby, but donor breast milk has many advantages over formula for very low birth-weight babies who are at the highest risk of necrotizing enterocolitis. Screening, pasteurizing, and storing milk is a major operation, so unfortunately milk banks are not available in every city.

Illness, exhaustion, and stress—all part of the premature experience—may affect milk supply. Babies who do not receive breast milk will be fed a formula designed specifically for premature babies. Formulas are as close a replica of breast milk as possible. Most are milk based and contain important nutrients such as DHEA and omega-3 fatty acids to promote development of the eyes and the nervous system. There are many different premature formulas, and the medical team will match one to your baby's specific nutritional needs.

12

Gastrointestinal Problems in the NICU

The gastrointestinal tract is a complex organ that starts at the mouth and ends at the anus. Though fully formed by the end of the first trimester, it's not fully operational until close to term. A healthy GI tract requires:

- **Rhythmic, organized contractions of the bowel,** also called **peristalsis,** to propel the contents of the bowel through the GI tract.
- **Intact lining of the bowel.** This absorbs nutrients, provides enzymes that digest milk, and offers a physical barrier against bacteria and toxins.
- **Healthy bacteria.** The GI tract is unique because interaction with bacteria is essential. Beneficial bacteria help eliminate toxins and keep dangerous bacteria at bay. Babies acquire these good bacteria from their mothers during delivery.
- **Good blood flow.** Oxygen supplied by the bloodstream is essential for normal functioning of every organ.
- **Healthy secretions.** The bowel produces mucus, which provides another layer of protection. Mucus also contains special antibodies, disease-fighting substances that protect against bacteria and viruses.

Necrotizing Enterocolitis

Necrotizing enterocolitis (NEC) is a condition in which the fragile premature bowel is injured, causing bacteria to enter the bowel wall and multiply. This can cause inflammation, infection, and bleeding problems. While NEC can happen to term babies, a premature baby is at greater risk because the immature GI tract is more susceptible to injury. The risk of NEC is approximately 10 percent among babies less than 1,500 g (3 lbs, 5 oz) at birth. NEC is *very* serious—15 to 30 percent of affected babies will die.

Feeding has a complex role in NEC. Breast milk is associated with fewer cases of NEC—it's the easiest food to digest and contains many bacteria-fighting substances. However, there are circumstances in which formula is the only option. Advancing feeds too quickly, whether breast milk or formula, can also cause problems—but simply continuing central nutrition indefinitely is not an option, as lack of food is damaging to the intestines, and the special intravenous is a potential source of infection.

Other factors that contribute to NEC include:

- **Disorganized bowel motility,** which allows harmful bacteria to overgrow. Premature bowels may take a while before they function appropriately.
- **Overgrowth of abnormal bacteria in the bowel.** Abnormal bacteria may be acquired in the NICU. Other factors that contribute to abnormal bacteria include delivery by C-section and antibiotics.
- **Reduced blood flow,** which damages the delicate bowel lining, increasing vulnerability to injury.
- **Immature immune system.**

The peak incidence of NEC is 14 to 20 days after birth. All babies at risk should be closely monitored. One of the challenges in diagnosing NEC is that the early warning signs are not specific and it can be difficult to distinguish from infection and other medical problems. Findings that raise concern about NEC include:

- **Increasing apneas and/or bradycardias.**
- **Distended belly** due to sluggish intestines and inflammation. Abdominal girth should be checked daily until your baby is well past the risk of NEC.
- **Feeding intolerance,** meaning bloating after feeds or excessive undigested food in the stomach (high feeding residuals). Many premature babies have feeding intolerance due to poorly organized bowel motility, but most never develop NEC.
- **Temperature instability,** either too high or too low.

If NEC is suspected, feeds will be stopped and your baby's stool may be tested for blood. NEC is diagnosed by specific X-ray findings of the abdomen. NEC is treated by giving antibiotics and draining bowel secretions with a nasogastric (NG) or orogastric (OG) tube. Other treatments may be needed to support your baby, including a medication called *dopamine* to improve blood flow to the bowels, a ventilator to help with breathing, and blood transfusions.

While many babies respond well to this treatment, the condition may worsen for 20 to 40 percent of babies and the bowel may rupture, spilling harmful bacteria in the belly and bloodstream. This may require emergency surgery to repair the bowel or placement of a small tube to drain the infection if the baby is too small or sick for surgery. Because of this risk, a pediatric surgeon should be involved as soon as the diagnosis of NEC is confirmed by X-ray. Babies who need bowel surgery for NEC are very sick, and unfortunately only 50 percent will survive, which is why preventing NEC is so important.

Constipation

More than 48 to 72 hours between bowel movements is considered abnormal when your baby is in the NICU. The most common causes of constipation are:

- **Motility problems.** Intestinal contractions are not well organized so food moves less efficiently through the premature GI tract. This is the most common cause of constipation for premature babies.
- **Exclusive intravenous feeding** (central nutrition), as food is necessary to stimulate the intestines.
- **Meconium plug.** Meconium is the first stool a baby passes. It is dark, thick, and sticky and is made up of mucus, bile, swallowed cells, and amniotic fluid. A blockage may result if the meconium does not pass. This is a cause of constipation in the first week of life.
- **Infection** anywhere in the body can affect the normal functioning of the GI tract.
- **Necrotizing enterocolitis.**
- **Thyroid abnormalities.**
- **Scar tissue,** the results of recovery from necrotizing enterocolitis.

The treatment of constipation includes mechanically stimulating the rectum by wiping or by inserting a tiny glycerin suppository. This can trigger the muscles to contract and move stool along. If a meconium plug is diagnosed, it may be flushed out with an enema.

Reflux

Reflux, or **gastroesophageal reflux (GER),** is the backward flow of stomach contents into the esophagus (the tube that connects the mouth with the stomach). If the contents make it into the mouth, it's called spitting up, and if they are expelled from the mouth, it is vomiting.

When food is swallowed it passes down the esophagus and through a muscle called the lower esophageal sphincter (LES), which opens to allow food to pass into the stomach and then closes to keep food in the stomach. (See Figure 9.) In many babies, both term and premature, the muscle is not strong enough to contain the food in the stomach or lacks the coordination required to open and close at the right time. Therefore some reflux is normal—some studies show that healthy preterm babies can have more than 70 brief reflux events in 24 hours.

FIGURE 9: The Stomach

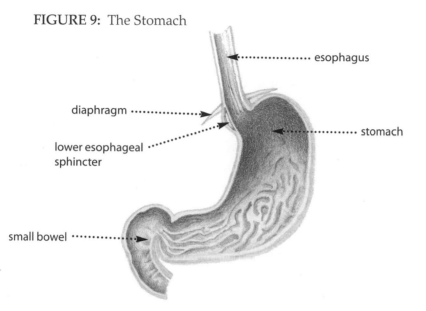

With time, all muscles strengthen and develop coordination, and the lower esophageal sphincter is no exception. For example, a term baby does not have enough muscle tone to lift her head for several months, but eventually the muscles in the neck get strong enough and the brain learns to control them. Among term babies, the function of the lower esophageal sphincter typically improves by six to 12 weeks; however, for a premature baby this maturation can take up to a year.

There are other factors that may contribute to reflux, including:

- **Slow stomach-emptying,** which leaves more food to reflux and more backward pressure on the LES.
- **Air swallowing** while eating. Uncoordinated, weaker muscles are less efficient, increasing air swallowing while eating. Swallowed air distends the stomach and increases pressure on the LES.
- **A hiatal hernia,** which is an opening in the diaphragm, the muscle that separates the stomach from the chest. A hiatal hernia allows part of the stomach to travel up into the chest. Not only is this uncomfortable, it makes it easier for food to reflux.

- **Breathing problems.** Breathing too fast or using too much energy to breathe makes reflux more likely.
- **A feeding tube.** Both an NG tube and an OG tube pass through the LES. While necessary for feeding, this tube may prevent the muscle between the esophagus and the stomach from closing completely.
- **Pyloric stenosis,** which is an abnormal tightening of the muscle (the pyloric sphincter) that controls the passage of food from the stomach to the intestines. When this muscle is too tight, food cannot pass through and is eventually vomited out the nose or mouth with force (projectile vomiting).

Almost every premature baby has some reflux, it's only a concern if there are significant symptoms or problems, such as:

- **Excessive irritability and/or back arching within an hour after feeds.** This is due to discomfort from the pressure and/or acid refluxing into the esophagus.
- **Apnea** or pauses in breathing may occur when a large amount of food is vomited.
- **Pneumonia** can occur if the vomited food particles are inhaled into the lungs.
- **Poor weight gain** may result if excessive amounts of food are vomited or if your baby has difficulty eating due to reflux.
- **Disorganized eating or an oral aversion.** The association of discomfort with eating can derail the transition from tube feeds to bottle. Your baby may turn her head or push away during attempts at eating. This can lead to more air swallowing, which further compounds the problem.

Until recently many doctors and researchers surmised that bradycardia within an hour of a meal could be the result of gastroesophageal reflux. However, there is new research emerging that questions the association between the two, so the idea that reflux causes bradycardia is controversial.

Victor's reflux started about 32 weeks adjusted age, as he was transitioning from continuous to bolus feeds. He fussed, arched his back, and was in agony. He was placed on his stomach, the head of his incubator elevated, but still he was in pain. I could set my watch by his bradycardia episodes, 45 minutes after a meal. Huge, swooping, downward strokes on the monitor as his heart rate dropped to 50 beats per minute. I would stimulate him, and up it would come, dropping again, and again, like riding the crests and troughs of perilous ocean waves.

We tried an angled bottle to reduce air swallowing, but no change. Acid-blockers did nothing. I even learned acupressure, but nothing helped. Perhaps there was a small improvement with thickened feeds, although by this time we were six weeks into the whole misadventure and it's entirely possible that time helped more than anything.

I finally cracked. I stormed up to the doctors and demanded, "Something has to be done."

Just the look on the doctor's face made me suddenly realize that if there were an effective therapy, it would already have been prescribed. I accepted there was nothing to do but wait, keep Victor as comfortable as possible, and watch for complications.

From then on I fed Oliver first so I could hold Victor after meals. I laid him face down on my stomach, as upright as possible, and just hugged him. We were like two lost souls clinging together, bobbing up and down in that bradycardial ocean. The reflux didn't stop, but the bradycardia gradually became less profound. Whether it was the touch therapy or time, I'll never know, but sometimes all you can do is try to weather the storm.

Almost all premature babies experience reflux, but not all reflux causes problems. In addition, other medical conditions can produce the same symptoms as reflux, so it can be difficult to determine symptoms that are reflux related and those that are not.

Tests can determine if reflux is present, but they don't indicate if reflux is actually the cause of the symptoms. Tests can be useful to rule out other conditions that may mimic reflux. If your baby has continued vomiting, difficulties gaining weight, or other reflux-related complications, your doctors may consider one or more of the following:

- **A pH probe test.** A small tube is inserted down the nose into the stomach. The tube measures acid levels at two points in the esophagus for 24 hours. In conjunction with heart rate and oxygen saturation monitoring this test may help determine if symptoms are associated with reflux.

- **A barium swallow** (also called an **upper GI series**). During this procedure, X-rays are taken while your baby drinks barium from a bottle (if your baby is unable to eat, the barium is given by a feeding tube.) The X-rays tell your baby's doctors if there are physical problems with the esophagus or stomach (such as a hiatal hernia) that may be contributing to reflux, vomiting, or feeding problems. A barium swallow is not a test for reflux.

- **An ultrasound** to look for pyloric stenosis if the vomiting is projectile and occurring with almost every meal.

As most premature babies eventually outgrow their reflux, the goal is to try to reduce discomfort and prevent complications while muscles improve in strength and coordination. Non-medication options may be considered first, such as:

- **Reviewing medications** to make sure they are not aggravating the condition. The most common drug in the NICU that aggravates reflux is caffeine.

- **Smaller, more frequent feeds.**

- **Burping frequently during feeds,** typically every 15 to 30 ml ($^1/_2$ to 1 oz), to reduce pressure buildup.

- **Keeping upright for 30 to 60 minutes after a feed.**

- **Keeping your baby on her stomach as much as possible,** which improves digestion. Lying on the stomach increases the risk of sudden infant death syndrome (SIDS); however, babies are closely monitored in the NICU, so in *this* environment it is safe.

- **Thickening feeds** to help food stay in the stomach. The best option is adding a product called *SimplyThick*, a thickening gel made with xanthum gum, to the feeds. The other option is to add oatmeal or rice cereal (generally 1 tsp per 30 ml of milk or formula). Thickened feeds are harder to suck through a nipple; if a fast-flow nipple is not working, the nurses will show you how to crosscut a nipple (make a small nick with a razor to slightly enlarge the hole). The downside to thickened feeds is slow digestion. If there is no improvement after two weeks, then thickened feeds should be stopped.

- **Transplyloric feeds.** A transpyloric tube (chapter 11) delivers food to the upper intestine, decreasing reflux from the stomach to the esophagus.

If symptoms due to reflux are severe and conservative options are not helping, medications may be required. All medications have risks, so it is important to balance the potential benefit against the severity of the symptoms. Medications take two to four weeks to work, so pay close attention to symptoms—keep a diary to track weight, irritability and discomfort, apnea episodes, and vomiting. Anti-reflux medications do not appear to help bradycardia associated with feedings. If there is no improvement after a four-week trial, then the medication is not helping. The two types of medications for reflux are:

- **Medications to reduce stomach acid** so the refluxed stomach contents are less irritating. There are two options, H2 blockers and proton pump inhibitors (PPIs). They both work well, although proton pump inhibitors are more effective at blocking acid. (See Table 1.) There is more experience with H2 blockers in premature babies, so most doctors will recommend starting with one of these drugs, but switch to a PPI if the symptoms persist despite therapy. The biggest concern with acid-blockers in the hospital is the increased risk of bloodstream infections because these medications change the balance of good bacteria in the intestine.
- **Medications to improve bowel contractions** so the stomach will empty more efficiently, leaving less stomach contents to reflux. The two options are *rantidine* (which is also an acid-blocker, so it can do double duty both lowering acid levels and improving

TABLE 1: Acid-Blocking Medications

Type of medication	Generic name	Brand name
H2 blocker	ranitidine*	Zantac
H2 blocker	cimetidine	Tagamet
Proton pump inhibitor	lansoprazole	Prevacid
Proton pump inhibitor	omeprazole	Prilosec, Zegrid
Proton pump inhibitor	esomeprazole	Nexium
Proton pump inhibitor	pantoprazole	Protonix
Proton pump inhibitor	rabeprazole	AcipHex

*Ranitidine has fewer side effects than cimetidine

contractions) and *metoclopramide (Reglan). Metoclopramide* can help some babies with slow stomach-emptying, but in the average premature baby with reflux no studies have shown it to be effective. It can make your baby sleepier, which may affect her ability to eat. *Metoclopramide* also has a black box warning from the Food and Drug Administration (FDA), which is an extra alert system to remind both providers and parents that it can cause **tardive dyskinesia,** a condition involving abnormal movements, tremors, and stiffness. These can almost always be immediately reversed with the antihistamine *diphenhydramine (Benadryl).* Permanent tardive dyskinesia is very rare in a baby taking the medication for a few months. If your baby is severely affected by reflux and there is evidence of slow stomach-emptying or the only other option is surgery, then a three- to four-week trial of *metoclopramide* is reasonable.

In some severe cases, surgery may be indicated. As reflux almost always gets better with time, surgery is only for babies who have complications that preclude waiting, such as pneumonia or problems gaining weight. Additional tests are necessary if surgery is considered. (See chapter 24.)

13

Vision and Hearing

Vision and Your Premature Baby

All of the structures required for vision are present by 22 weeks, but there are still major developmental milestones that must occur for normal vision to develop:

- **A special network of blood vessels must develop in the back of the retina.** The retina lines the inside of the eye and contains cells that change light signals into electrical energy.
- **The nervous system must mature,** meaning both the nerves that carry signals to the brain (the optic nerves) and the connections within the brain itself.
- **The eyelids must open.** They are fused shut until 25 to 27 weeks. Your baby can see when her eyes open, although it's unknown how well.

While the darkness of the womb stimulates development of the visual system, exposure to bright hospital lights in the NICU does not contribute to eye disease or visual impairment. However, the bili lights used to treat jaundice may be damaging, so protective eyewear is necessary even if your baby's eyes are still closed, as her fused eyelids only filter out some of this potentially harmful light.

Even though the lights of the NICU are not damaging, dark, quiet time for rest and sleep is essential. It gives the nervous system downtime to develop and improves both sleep patterns and weight gain. While your baby is still in an incubator, a quilt or blanket is used to block out light during quiet time. When your baby graduates to an open crib, the best option is an area of the NICU where the lights can be dimmed at night.

Retinopathy of Prematurity (ROP)

Retinopathy of prematurity (ROP) is a disorder involving the growth of abnormal blood vessels in the retina. It is triggered by exposure to higher oxygen levels before 35 weeks. The abnormal blood vessels are fragile and can break, causing bleeding, or they may overgrow and become thick, then pull on the retina and cause it to detach from the inside of the eye. This can lead to blindness.

ROP affects 15,000 premature infants a year in the United States. Most cases resolve without treatment, but 1 to 2 percent of babies less than 1,500 g (3 lbs, 5 oz) at birth will become blind, and many more babies will be left with some type of visual impairment. Screening for ROP is critical, and an early intervention by an ophthalmologist (eye specialist) can help prevent this damage.

Risk factors for ROP include:

- **The degree of prematurity.** The more premature, the greater the risk; 83 percent of babies born before 28 weeks will develop some degree of ROP.
- **Birth weight.** Babies who weigh less than 1,000 g (2 lbs, 3 oz) are at greatest risk.
- **Need for oxygen,** because high levels of oxygen trigger the growth of abnormal blood vessels.
- **Other medical problems.**

ROP is divided into stages, from 0 to 5, depending on the condition of the blood vessels and the retina. (See Table 1.)

TABLE 1: Stages of ROP and Need for Intervention

Stage ROP	Outcome
Stage 0 Immature blood vessels	May progress to ROP or may develop normally
Stage 1 Mildly abnormal vessels	90% resolve, 10% progress
Stage 2 Moderately abnormal vessels	90% resolve, 10% progress
Stage 3 Severely abnormal vessels	50% resolve spontaneously, 50% need treatment
Stage 4 Partially detached retina	Need treatment
Stage 5 Detached retina	Need treatment

All babies less than 1,500 g at birth should be screened for ROP, and babies weighing 1,500 to 2,000 g (3 lbs, 5 oz to 4 lbs, 7 oz) who have experienced significant medical problems should also be screened. The timing of your baby's first eye exam will depend on her gestational age. (See Table 2.) Eye exams are not performed immediately after birth because it takes time for the abnormal blood vessels to develop. In addition, your baby must be able to tolerate the exam without having her heart rate or oxygen levels drop.

The exam for ROP is performed in the NICU by an ophthalmologist who is either a pediatric or a retina specialist. Drops to anesthetize (numb) the eyes and dilate the pupils are given by the nurses 30 minutes before the exam. While the nurse swaddles and holds your baby, the ophthalmologist re-applies the numbing drops and then uses an instrument called an eye speculum to hold the eyelids open. The ophthalmologist evaluates the retina with a hand lens (a very powerful magnifying glass) and a headlamp. It looks very uncomfortable with the eye speculum in place, but the eye drops help, as does a sugarcoated pacifier.

Eye exams are performed every one to three weeks until normal vessels have spread throughout the retina and there is no more risk of ROP. Normal blood vessels may not fully develop until several weeks after discharge from the NICU.

TABLE 2: Timing of Initial Eye Exam for ROP (adapted from *Screening Examination of Premature Infants for Retinopathy of Prematurity*, American Academy of Pediatrics policy statement, 2006)

Gestational age at birth	Age of initial eye exam for ROP	
	Unadjusted age in weeks	Adjusted age (Weeks since birth)
22	31	9
23	31	8
24	31	7
25	31	6
26	31	5
27	31	4
28	32	4
29	33	4
30	34	4
31	34	2–3
32	34	1–2

I sat through every procedure in the NICU, but I confided to the nurses that I didn't think I could make it through the eye exams. Not only does a retina exam look uncomfortable (even for adults), but eyeballs gross me out. Yes, I am a surgeon. And yes, I do plenty of stomach-turning procedures, but the eye is another thing altogether. I can't even watch my husband take out his contact lenses.

The nurses explained it looks worse than it really is. The biggest issue is that the babies must be very still so the doctor can properly evaluate the entire retina. The nurses know the routine so well that they can help the eye doctor make the exam as fast as possible.

I am a big proponent of staying by the bedside for procedures, but I also believe babies can pick up on a parent's mood. For me, watching a procedure where I couldn't be involved or even hold a finger for comfort was just going to be too much. I did feel guilty about not being at the bedside for the eye exams, but in the end it was the right thing to do. We all have different limits, and that's okay.

Treatment is indicated if Stage 3 ROP does not resolve, and always for Stage 4 and 5. Therapy for ROP in these circumstances reduces the risk of blindness. A laser is used to burn the edge of the retina, the area where the abnormal blood vessels have yet to appear. This peripheral part of the retina is actually stimulating the growth of the abnormal vessels, and when it's destroyed the abnormal vessels stop growing and eventually disappear. This treatment is a trade-off. It damages some peripheral vision in an attempt to preserve the more important central vision. Even with treatment many babies will be nearsighted and need glasses. Cryotherapy (freezing) of the retina is sometimes used; however, there is a higher incidence of nearsightedness after cryotherapy as opposed to laser therapy.

Some babies can have the laser surgery performed at their bedside with sedation while others need to go to the operating room. The decision to go to the operating room depends on many factors, including the availability of the equipment in the NICU, how much medication is needed to keep your baby comfortable and immobile for the procedure, and underlying medical stability, such as apneas and bradycardias. The doctors will try to do the procedure without putting your baby on a ventilator, because each time a premature baby goes back on a ventilator, the risk of lung damage increases.

Laser therapy for ROP takes about one hour for each eye. The laser is directed through the pupil to the retina, which lines the inside of the eye. The eyes and eyelids may be red and swollen for a few days. Eye drops are required for seven days and an exam is repeated no later than a week; if the response is unsatisfactory, another treatment may be required.

If there has been retinal detachment, additional therapies are needed. One procedure is called a **scleral buckle,** which involves placing a silicone band around the eye, like a belt, and tightening it to flatten the retina against the back of the eye. The other procedure is a **vitrectomy,** only performed for stage 4 or 5 ROP, where the scar tissue in the retina is removed, releasing the tension on the retina and allowing it to lie flat again.

Cortical Visual Impairment

Cortical visual impairment (CVI) may occur when the occipital lobe, the part of the brain that interprets electrical signals from the eyes, is injured. The incidence of CVI is 1 percent to 3 percent among premature babies, and the risk is highest among those with lower birth weights. The most common causes of CVI are lack of oxygen (hypoxemia) or insufficient blood flow to the brain (ischemia), but other causes include hydrocephalus (excessive cerebrospinal fluid in the brain), hypoglycemia (low blood sugar), and infections.

CVI is difficult to diagnose initially, as the eye exam is normal. It is usually suspected when an ultrasound shows abnormalities in the occipital lobe. An MRI of the brain is needed to gather more information, but it cannot predict the degree of visual impairment. Significant recovery can occur, and most children with abnormal scans have some vision, although 10 percent with abnormal scans are completely blind. If only one side of the brain is injured, color perception may be preserved, as both sides of the brain interpret color.

If an ultrasound or MRI has raised concerns about CVI, you should follow up with both a pediatric ophthalmologist and a neurologist after discharge home from the NICU.

Hearing

The incidence of hearing loss for babies who spend more than two days in an NICU is approximately 2.5 percent. This is 10 times the risk of hearing impairment compared with a baby born at term.

All of the parts for hearing have developed by 24 weeks, and by 28 weeks the auditory pathways are mature enough that in the uterus a baby consistently responds to sound by moving, blinking, and increasing heart rate. At 28 weeks a baby's hearing is developed enough to hear a sound of 40 dB or louder. (See Table 3.) After that, the ability to detect softer sounds improves as the pregnancy advances, and by 42 weeks hearing is the same as in an adult.

More than one factor may be involved in hearing loss, so it's often difficult to identify a specific cause. The three types of hearing loss and causes are listed in Table 4.

TABLE 3: Decibels (dB) of Common Sounds

Sound in dB	Activity
13.5	Threshold for hearing
20	Whisper
40	Refrigerator humming
60	Normal conversation
70	Vacuum cleaner
85	Need to raise voice to be heard in a conversation
90	Power lawn mower

TABLE 4: Types and Causes of Hearing Loss

Type of hearing loss	What it is	cause
Conductive	Sound vibrations are not transmitted correctly to the inner ear	Abnormality of ear, ear canal, eardrum, or bones of middle ear
Sensorineural	Damage to the hair cells in the inner ear that translate sound vibrations into electrical energy	Infection Genetics Medications Noise Birth defects involving the inner ear
Central	Damage to the nerve that transmits the electrical energy to the brain, or damage to the area in the brain that processes signals into sound	High bilirubin levels in blood Hypoxia (low oxygen levels) Hypotension (low blood pressure) Intraventricular hemorrhage

I talked to my boys a lot. I was careful to observe quiet time while their incubators were covered with a quilt, but I could hardly wait for their day to begin; I felt like a little girl anxiously waiting for the candy store to open. While I changed their diapers and took their temperatures, I told them about our dogs and what had happened at home the night before, as if my Crock-Pot and *The Tonight Show* was a grand tale. I also told them how strong they were and how I was surprised by how much I needed them.

It's hard to chatter on for weeks on end without any feedback. And then, seven weeks into their stay in the NICU, it happened. I walked in one morning and started talking with Oliver's nurse. I was standing behind his crib. All he could see was the nurse, but he was hearing my voice. The nurse laughed, "He's looking for you."

And he was. I peered around and saw his face before he saw mine. Confused by the mismatch of face and voice, his little eyes were looking all around as if to say, "You're not *my* mama." And then the moment his little features found my face I saw his furrowed brow relax and his eyes changed. It was as if he'd screamed, "Mama!"

I probably told a hundred people that day that Oliver, my son, knew my voice.

Effects of Noise Exposure in the NICU

People generally find sounds between 60 and 90 dB annoying, and sounds louder than 90 dB damage the hair cells in the inner ear and can lead to sensorineural hearing loss. Noise can adversely affect blood pressure, heart rate, and oxygen levels. It may also disrupt growth and development. Some babies with sensory processing disorders may be extra sensitive to even low levels of noise. Finally, noise is distracting, and doctors, nurses, and the rest of the medical team function best with the least amount of distractions.

For all these reasons, it's recommended that NICUs keep the background noise to less than 45 dB (between a whisper and normal conversation) and adopt a policy of individualized environmental care (IEC), which means optimizing the environment for a premature baby. Examples of IEC include draining water that accumulates in the ventilator (to reduce

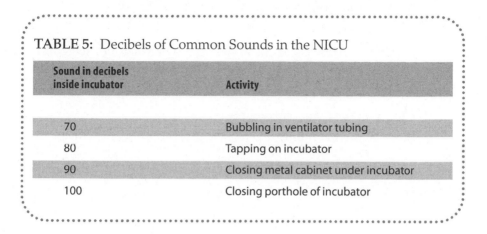

TABLE 5: Decibels of Common Sounds in the NICU

Sound in decibels inside incubator	Activity
70	Bubbling in ventilator tubing
80	Tapping on incubator
90	Closing metal cabinet under incubator
100	Closing porthole of incubator

the noise from bubbling), soft shoes, no tapping or writing on the incubator, opening and closing incubator doors carefully, limiting bedside conversation to a normal or low voice, and covering the incubator with a quilt or blanket as a muffler. (See Table 5 for common sounds in the NICU.) Prolonged periods of quiet, especially at night, are also needed.

Some sounds are beneficial, especially a parent's voice. During pregnancy a baby hears her mother's voice best. (They also hear Dad's voice, just not as well.) When a baby is born prematurely, talking or singing while she is awake allows her to still hear these important sounds and helps the developing nervous system. It is also comforting to hear the same sounds over and over, especially when associated with a reassuring touch. Even though your baby may have the most amazing nurse in the world, a nurse is there for three days at a time and then is gone for several days. A parent's voice provides consistency and stability.

Sensory Processing Disorder and Noise

Some babies in the NICU can become jittery or stressed in response to sounds. They may react with concerning changes in heart rate, blood pressure, and oxygen level. These are signs that noise is over-stimulating the nervous system and should not be ignored. Interventions can help to minimize these abnormal responses, including:

- **A quieter location** in the NICU.
- **Headphones** playing soft classical music or a recording of Mom or Dad's voice. Blocking out all sounds is a bad idea, but switching a disquieting noise for a pleasing sound can be helpful.
- **Re-introducing sounds gradually** when appropriate with the help of an occupational therapist.
- **Parents' involvement,** which is the most soothing presence.

Hearing Tests Before Discharge

To allow the auditory system to mature sufficiently, testing is not performed until 34 weeks. There are two types of hearing tests; both are painless and are best performed while your baby is sleeping or eating, because movement and crying can give inaccurate results:

- **Transient evoked otoacoustic emission (TEOAE)** involves placing a device in the ear that emits a sound. When hair cells in the inner ear bend in response to sound waves, they create a different sound that is detected by a microphone in the device.
- **Automated auditory brainstem response (AABR)** involves headphones that deliver a series of soft clicks to the ears, and electrodes on the forehead and neck that evaluate the brain's response to the sound.

These are screening tests and do have false positives, meaning your baby does not pass the test but the test is incorrect and your baby can hear just fine. As many as 30 percent of initial hearing tests can be incorrectly positive, and this is more likely if your baby was agitated or crying during the exam.

If a test is positive, it's repeated about a week later, usually with the other testing method. If your baby passes the second test, there is no need to worry. If both tests are positive for possible hearing loss, then follow-up with an audiologist (hearing specialist) is essential, as 80 percent of these babies will have some kind of hearing loss.

PART THREE

The Mind–Body Connection

14

Emotional Health

Prematurity takes the fears and concerns of new parents to a different level. In addition to all the typical pregnancy and post-delivery concerns, parents with a premature baby may worry about whether their baby will ever learn to breast-feed, how they will manage with home oxygen, or if their baby will ever learn to walk. Some worry that their baby might not make it through the night. For many parents, the anxiety, stress, and worry that accompany prematurity persist for years. While these fears and stressors are unavoidable, if you proactively deal with these emotions, you will be more resilient.

Grief

Grief is a normal response to loss. It's an intensely painful emotional and physical experience. You may grieve the loss of a perfect pregnancy, the loss of a normal birth experience, the effects of prematurity on your baby, or the most intense grief of all, the loss of a baby.

While everyone grieves differently, the most common symptoms are intense sadness, difficulty sleeping, and loss of appetite. Other feelings include yearning, disbelief, anger, frustration, and helplessness. Many people also have physical symptoms such as pain, shortness of breath, and exhaustion.

Grief is not linear. It's a dynamic process with good days and not so good days. It is much harder at the beginning when the loss is still very raw, but as the mind starts assimilating the loss into the framework of life, the pain gradually lessens and the bad days become less frequent and less intense.

Most people will notice improvement in symptoms, but not complete resolution, within a few months. There may be episodes when the symptoms resurface with an unbelievable rawness, triggered by specific events such as your due date, a friend's baby shower, or the birthday of a deceased child. This grief may be as intense and painful as the initial emotion, but will resolve much quicker.

I never really understood despair until my boys were born. It's true that life was better when they came home, but I was having difficulty getting my brain around "Why?" I was angry, sad, and resentful. I threw myself into their medical needs because it was easier than opening the Pandora's box of my emotions.

One night, as I lay on the couch wrapped in a blanket of grief and self-pity, I was flipping channels on the TV and stopped for some unknown reason at *The Tonight Show*. Jay Leno was interviewing Nicole Kidman and the conversation turned to her divorce from Tom Cruise. It was clearly very painful for her to discuss. She mentioned how she had problems accepting the loss. When asked how she had managed to cope, she repeated advice she received from her father. "It is what it is. It is not what it was meant to be, but it is what it is."

At that moment she was not a Hollywood star, but a fragile woman who had been deeply hurt, sharing an intimate father-daughter moment. I was moved by her frailty and candor.

Her father's advice was simple, brilliant, and insightful, because dealing with tragedy is about accepting a new reality. We are meant to move forward, not dwell in the past. It's only when you accept a situation that you can learn how to adapt, which is essential for both emotional and physical survival.

That night I repeated out loud, "It is what it is," and I drew strength from hearing the words. I repeated them over and over, each time feeling a little bit better. In the past six years I have repeated them again and again, sometimes out loud and sometimes to myself. These five words have become my mantra, and they are truly words to live by.

The grieving process is influenced by personality, culture, religion, and spiritual beliefs, as well as previous experiences. Grief does not require medical therapy, although if you're having trouble sleeping, talk with your doctor about a sleep aid. Never underestimate the importance of a good night's sleep in your body's ability to heal.

There is no right or wrong way to grieve, although most people feel better when they open up about their feelings. Some ideas include:

- **Journaling** your thoughts and fears, because some feelings are too complex, private, or raw to say a loud.
- **A baby book** to create positive memories. Milestones may be different, such as getting off the ventilator, reaching 1,000 g (2 lbs, 3 oz), or taking a first bottle. These are amazing joy-filled moments that should be celebrated.
- **Support from another parent** who has experienced prematurity. Someone who has been there can understand and validate your emotions. Even being in touch by phone or e-mail with another parent a few times a week can make a big difference.
- **Religious or spiritual support.**
- **Talking with a therapist or grief counselor** who can offer you specific, proactive ways to address grief.
- **Addressing your physical needs.** Sleeping, eating right, and exercising are essential for both physical and emotional health. Exercise also releases natural endorphins that can impart a sense of well-being.
- **Embracing your feelings.** It's okay to cry, laugh, or be angry. Letting emotions out is better than keeping them bottled up.
- **Reading about other people's experiences** with prematurity or other challenges. Read a memoir. People don't write about their happy, perfect, stress-free lives, they write about coping with a tragedy or a difficult time. (There is a reason memoirs are so popular!)

I was the queen of avoiding triggers. I refused to sign up for the Mothers of Multiples club because I couldn't bear the thought of seeing triplets. I hated being around strangers because inevitably someone would approach cooing, "What beautiful twins." I was always flummoxed. Do I respond, "Actually, they are triplets?" and bear the pain of the explanation for a stranger who doesn't *really* want to know? Do I respond with the appropriate niceties and say, "Yes, they are twins," letting the wound rip open and fester once again? Sometimes I could avoid it with a simple nod. However, there was often a follow-up question, like a one-two punch in the boxer's ring: "Who is the eldest?" I wanted to shout, "Neither!" but usually I would lie and point to Oliver.

Then my mother-in-law came to visit. She had lost her middle child, my husband's younger brother David, when he was 15. When a neighbor of ours asked her how many children she had, without batting an eye she answered, "Four who are with me and one who is in heaven." I was astounded and so proud of her at the same time.

So I started the same approach. When people asked if my boys were twins, I responded, "No, they are triplets, but their oldest brother did not come home from the hospital." Sometimes it was clear they didn't *really* want to hear it, but I didn't care. I needed to say it. I had to hear it, accept it, and deal with it.

Gradually being around people and answering questions became easier and easier, but I still avoided triplets. Then some years later I came face to face with an unexpected set: triplet ogres at the end of *Shrek the Third*. Much to my surprise, I laughed just like everyone else.

- **Be proactive about grief triggers.** At some point these triggers must be faced, so it's a good idea to develop some helpful coping strategies. This is where a therapist can be helpful.
- **Reduce stress.** Stress is emotionally distracting and makes every problem seem worse. Try to lighten your load by simplifying other situations.
- **Control anxiety before it controls you.** Anxiety stirs the emotional pot. There are excellent mental and physical exercises to help

you regain control (see chapter 15, Medical Mindfulness); some people may need a medication to treat anxiety.

Baby Blues

Some mothers have intense episodes of sadness, worry, fear, anger, or anxiety after childbirth. They may cry for no reason or have trouble eating and sleeping and wonder if they are really prepared for parenting. These feelings are called the baby blues, and they affect 70 to 80 percent of women. The baby blues are caused by the physical, emotional, and hormonal upheaval of delivering a baby.

The baby blues share some symptoms with depression. However, unlike depression, the emotions of the baby blues do not permeate every waking thought, but come and go in waves. The baby blues usually improve within two weeks.

Postpartum Depression

Postpartum depression typically starts two weeks to two months after delivery. It affects 15 to 20 percent of women who deliver at term and 10 percent of fathers/partners; it's more common among parents with a premature baby.

This type of depression has some of the same symptoms as grief and the baby blues, such as sadness, fatigue, trouble sleeping, anxiety, and changes in appetite. However, these symptoms are more intense and pervasive and affect everyday life. It's possible to be distracted from grief by moments of happiness or pleasure, but not from depression. Symptoms that suggest depression include:

- **Intense despair.**
- **Severe guilt.**
- **Impaired concentration.**
- **Thoughts of suicide or a preoccupation with dying.**

- Feelings of hopelessness or worthlessness.
- Slow speech and body movements.
- Seeing or hearing things that aren't there.
- **Being overwhelmed by daily activities** such as getting out of bed, getting dressed, pumping breast milk, or visiting the NICU.

Postpartum depression is not a sign of weakness and it certainly isn't anyone's fault. It's a real medical problem and the result of biochemical changes in the brain. Factors that contribute to postpartum depression include:

- **Changes in hormones after delivery.**
- **Underlying vulnerability.** Some people are genetically more susceptible to depression.
- **Stress,** both physical and emotional, affects brain chemistry. In addition to the stress of a complicated pregnancy and the NICU, parents with premature babies experience more general life stressors, such as relationship conflict and financial pressures.
- **Disturbed sleep** affected by long hours at the hospital and worry. This has a profoundly negative effect on brain chemistry.
- **Worry** about your baby's health problems as well as finances, job stability, and how your other children are coping.
- **Lack of support.** Parents with babies in the intensive care unit often have no one with whom to share their experiences and fears.
- **Lack of time to adjust to birth.**
- **Guilt.**
- **Disrupted bonding.**
- **Grief.**
- **Breast-feeding problems.**
- **Loss of control.**
- **Negative interactions with health care providers.**

Recognizing and treating postpartum depression is essential. Depression causes emotional pain, affects your physical health, and can even lead to suicide. Depression also affects your baby—children who grow up around a depressed parent are more likely to develop physical, emotional, and behavioral problems. Your emotional health affects your baby in so many ways.

Ask your OB/GYN, nurse practitioner, or midwife about depression. There are questionnaires that are very effective screening tools. The main treatment options for depression are therapy (with a psychologist or counselor) and antidepressants. An OB/GYN may feel comfortable prescribing antidepressants or may refer you to a psychiatrist, a doctor who specializes in treating depression and other mood disorders. Needing medications is not a sign of weakness. Many medical conditions require medication. If antidepressants are recommended, the prescribing doctor should check with your neonatologist to make sure the drug is compatible with breast-feeding.

Some people have difficulty accepting depression as a real medical condition or that they need help. Many parents feel "If my baby were healthy and at home I wouldn't be depressed." While that might be true, no matter how many times you wish things were different, prematurity will not magically disappear, and neither will the biochemical changes that cause depression.

All of the approaches already discussed for grief may also help with depression. Other suggestions include:

- **Set a schedule.** Many people feel better with a routine; it restores a small amount of order to an otherwise chaotic situation. Include showering, scheduled breaks, and meals. Set aside time every day for a few minutes of self-care. (See chapter 15, Medical Mindfulness.)
- **Exercise.** Any activity that increases heart rate also releases endorphins, which have a very positive effect on mood.
- **Sleep.** Nap when your baby sleeps, and if you have help at home, divide the night into shifts so you both get some uninterrupted sleep.

Post-Traumatic Stress Disorder (PTSD)

PTSD is a collection of persistent physical and emotional reactions to a traumatic, scary, or otherwise negative experience. It's a normal response to an abnormal situation. It is not depression, but some people with PTSD also suffer from depression.

Most people associate PTSD with the trauma of war or an assault, like rape, but it can be triggered by any fear-inducing experience. PTSD affects 76 percent of mothers who deliver prematurely as well as a significant number of their partners.

The traumas of prematurity are not confined to the physical and emotional pain of delivery. Having your baby in the NICU causes a constant state of severe emotional stress. At the hospital you may witness the suffering of your baby, and when you're at home you worry that the next phone call will be devastating news. These traumas may continue for years if your baby has chronic health problems.

You also have fewer opportunities to work through your emotions and fears. Going to the hospital every day is physically and emotionally isolating. Even if you have the opportunity to share, it can be difficult because of perceived guilt, or family and friends who don't grasp the gravity of the situation or tire of hearing about the NICU and continued health problems.

You may have PTSD if you experience some of the following for more than a month:

- **Being haunted by an experience,** reliving it over and over again in memories, flashbacks, or nightmares.
- **Anxiety or panic** when exposed to reminders.
- **Avoiding reminders** of the trauma.
- **Feeling numb or detached** from others.
- **Difficulty sleeping.**
- **Difficulty concentrating.**
- **Feeling jumpy or on guard** all the time.

PTSD can have a negative impact on your baby's development. It also affects your well-being. There's no quick fix; however, acknowledging your feelings and that the physical symptoms are not "all in your head," but part of a real medical condition, can be helpful.

For many, a psychologist or psychiatrist who understands the disorder is an essential part of recovery. They can help you work through the unresolved trauma and reframe your emotional responses as well as provide tools to help you cope with anxiety and prevent panic attacks. Many parents also find respite talking with other parents who have experienced prematurity; having the support of someone who knows what you're going through is invaluable. Some parents who suffer from PTSD may need medications for anxiety, panic attacks, or depression.

Specific interventions that have proven useful for preventing PTSD include:

- **Talking about the traumatic experiences.** Your feelings need to be expressed.
- **Learning and practicing relaxation techniques.** (See chapter 15.)
- **Support from another parent with a premature baby.** Someone who has been there can validate your feelings and listen with a real understanding.
- **Support from therapist, social worker, or counselor.**
- **Solving concrete problems** like sick leave or child care for your child at home. Stress multiplies in an exponential fashion, so taking everything else off the table makes it easier for you to focus on the healing process.

15

Medical Mindfulness

Mind-body medicine is the idea that our thoughts and emotions influence physical health, and harnessing this connection improves both emotional and physical well-being.

Chemicals, such as neurotransmitters and hormones, send messages back and forth throughout the body. They're like keys on a keyboard—certain sequences and situations convey very different messages. It's this shared alphabet that is the very core of the mind-body connection and allows stress and anxiety, which affect neurotransmitters and hormones, to have a negative effect on every organ system, but especially on inflammation and the immune system.

Fortunately, this mind-body connection can be harnessed for a positive effect. Positive thoughts and emotional well-being promote the best chemical interactions in our bodies. Neurotransmitters and hormones that contribute to medical conditions can be altered with drugs, but we can also sneak in the back door with medical mindfulness, which is the practice of actively using thoughts and actions to create the most healing environment. For most conditions, the mind-body connection does not replace traditional Western medicine, but it's a wonderful complement and a way to optimize outcomes.

The mind-body connection applies to prematurity in three ways:

- **Your emotional health during pregnancy.** Pregnancy is the ultimate bonding experience—a physical connection with shared chemicals, hormones, and rhythms. *All* of these connections are important for a developing baby. Depression changes brain chemistry and affects hormones, doubling the risk of premature delivery. Depression, stress, and anxiety also lower birth weight.
- **A premature baby's stress response.** Babies are hard-wired to combat the stress of moving from the dark, warm uterus to the cold, harsh outside environment with self-soothing behavior, such as bringing their hands to their mouths and sucking. Premature babies are not only exposed to more physical stress, but because of nervous system immaturity and illness, they're less able to mount these protective responses. Prolonged exposure to stress can affect development of the nervous system and the immune system and can adversely influence many medical conditions.
- **Your emotional health after delivery.** Parents and premature babies develop important connections very quickly, which are essential for developing a healthy stress response and learning to organize behavior. Premature babies whose parents have higher stress levels are more likely to have abnormal levels of stress hormones themselves. This puts them at higher risk for colic, disturbed sleep patterns as well as feeding, behavior, and developmental problems.

The mind-body connection is an area where you can have a *major* impact on your premature baby's health. Optimizing your emotional health before and after delivery, reducing environmental stressors to which your baby is exposed, and helping your baby to develop a protective stress response will not only reduce your stress and help you feel more empowered, but will also create an optimal environment for your baby's health and development. Studies show that reducing parental stress has a positive effect on a premature baby, so if these techniques make you feel better, then in some way, large or small, your baby *has* benefited.

Medical Mindfulness Techniques for Parents

Mind-body techniques exercise both physical and emotional health. There are many different techniques, some more involved than others. To avoid getting overwhelmed, start at a comfortable level of personal engagement. Just as with any exercise program, you should get comfortable with the first level and progress as you feel the need. It requires practice to master many of these techniques, so take it slow. Try one or two of the Level 1 techniques every day, and then gradually add in others as your mood and emotions dictate. You don't want to get overwhelmed or worry that you're not relaxing hard enough!

Level 1

These are the simplest techniques and are universally beneficial. They require no special equipment or skills, yet have far-reaching effects.

- Practice **breath awareness.** When we stress and tense, we breathe with our chest muscles instead of breathing from the diaphragm (also called belly breathing). Chest breathing is shallow, less efficient, and tiring, and it contributes to the stress cycle. Deep belly breathing is a simple and effective tool for stopping a stressful moment in its tracks. What exactly is belly breathing? Look at how a young child takes a breath—their belly moves up and down. Now place your own hand on your belly. Is it rising with each breath? Slow and steady movements that cause your belly to rise and fall are the goal. Before you fall asleep, practice belly breathing for a few minutes. Several times during the day, stop what you're doing and practice these cleansing belly breaths for a few minutes. Any time you feel stressed, put your hand on your belly and focus on taking these deep, natural breaths.

- **Go for a 10-minute walk.** Exercise improves circulation, forces you to belly breathe, and releases endorphins (chemicals that make you feel better). Being outside and breathing fresh air is also very therapeutic. When your baby is in the hospital it's hard to leave, but think of it as therapy for both of you. Once you're at home your can bundle your baby up in the stroller and she can enjoy the walk as well, or have your partner give you 10 minutes alone to walk by yourself.

- **Make every effort to get enough sleep.** Sleep deprivation alters stress hormones. Sleep is a time when you're free from new stressors and your brain can process the stressful events of the day. It's better to have a good night's rest, even if it means spending fewer hours at the hospital, than to be around constantly, but harried and full of stress. *Taking care of yourself is not abandoning your baby— it's helping.* Once your baby comes home, forget the housework and make sure to sleep when your baby does. If there are two of you at night, consider shifts for nighttime feeding and diaper changes.

Tony brought me a journal a few days after I delivered. He meant it as a notebook to track my attempts at pumping breast milk. I was so stressed and sick I couldn't remember when I had last pumped, so he thought writing it down might help. In addition to the volume of milk and the times I pumped, I started writing random thoughts, and gradually words replaced the numbers. I was afraid to say many things, but I could write them. As time passed I would look back on what I had written. I could see how terrified I had been for my boys, maybe only a week before, and how I thought I would die from a broken heart, and yet we were all still here.

I still read these journals. I run my fingers over the writing as if it were Braille, and feeling the paper, worn with touch, I am instantly transported back to the NICU. I can feel the fear in my chest, hear the staccato of the machines, and smell the hospital. But I also remember the joy when I first held them, my elation when they gained weight, and the first time I gave them a bottle. It's tangible evidence of both the pain and the triumphs. It is our proof of strength.

- **Pay attention to your thoughts and feelings.** When you find your stress level rising, stop what you're doing. There is a lot of therapy in just pausing. The next step is to shift your focus away from what you cannot change, such as oxygen levels and infection, and focus on what you can influence, such as positive interactions with your baby or learning more about her condition.

Level 2

These techniques require only slightly more effort. Pick at least one activity and try to practice it three times a day. If that one doesn't seem to help, try another—some therapies are just a better fit. Like any medical therapy, you will not see benefit over night; it may take three or four weeks.

- **Affirmations** are positive statements that when repeated help combat negative thoughts and feelings by reprogramming the unconscious mind. Podcasts and CDs are available. Affirmations can also be read out loud—there are books, preprinted cards, and even services that will text affirmations to your cell phone. Another option is to buy a pack of 3 × 5 cards and create your own affirmations. Some examples include, "I will let go of expectations," "I am strong and courageous," and "I will share my inner strength with my baby."

- **Body scans** are a way to gauge your level of muscle tension, which is a physical manifestation of stress. Starting at your head and gradually working your way down your body to your toes, pay close attention to pain or tension in each body part as you go, and make a conscious effort to relax each part as you focus on it. If you can't tell if an area is tense, actively tighten the muscle as much as you can and then relax—that feeling of letting go is what you are aiming for. Start with your scalp and then move down to your forehead, cheeks, lips, chin, and so on. Keep your eyes closed or open and scan your body slowly—it might take a minute or so on each body part. When you've done a full body scan once or twice, it will become apparent where you carry your tension and stress. (Forehead, neck, shoulders, and back are the biggest culprits.) Do a full body scan at least once a day and incorporate mini-scans of problem spots two or three times during the day, or any time you feel your stress level rising.

- **Guided imagery** is the practice of listening to suggestions that help your conscious and unconscious mind become more connected with your body. This can help with healing, body awareness, and stress reduction. One example is to let your imagination take you to a beach—focus on the feel and smell of the sand, air, and water. Guided imagery is best done in a quiet room, so you can tune out distractions. You can work one-on-one with a therapist or instructor, look for specific scripts online or in books, or listen to a CD or podcast. Links for free downloads of guided imagery (as well as affirmations) are available at www.preemieprimer.com.
- **Keeping your hands busy.** Start a craft, such as scrapbooking a baby book. Celebrate with pictures and record your thoughts. Knitting, crocheting, and sewing are also excellent stress relievers.

Level 3

These techniques are more involved because they need more practice or the help of a therapist or instructor.

- **Meditation** is the practice of paying attention to one thought to bring about a state of calm and relaxation. Normally you are bombarded with many thoughts and stressors, and this is even more pronounced if your baby is sick. By focusing on one positive thought or emotion you can remove the negative effects of intrusive thoughts and stressful situations.
- **Yoga** is the practice of creating physical and mental balance. It involves a combination of poses that develop strength and flexibility, and meditative thoughts. Yoga may be practiced with an instructor at the gym or studio or at home with the help of a book, TV show, or DVD.

- **Qi Gong** and **Tai Chi** are traditional Chinese movements that can be very helpful in developing physical and mental awareness as well as reducing stress.
- **Biofeedback** is a way to develop awareness and control of your body functions by paying attention to physical signals normally not in your conscious awareness, such as heart rate and muscle spasm. Because these physical signals are affected by stress, learning to control them through biofeedback is a way to reduce the effect of stress on your body. Biofeedback can be performed with a licensed therapist who uses equipment to provide visual signals, but it can also be tried at home. When you feel anxious or stressed, check your heart rate at your wrist for 30 seconds and make note of how fast your heart is beating. Keep your fingers on your pulse so you are feeling your heart rate in real time, think calming thoughts, and focus on things that are slow. It even helps to think or whisper happy thoughts or affirmations about the positive effects of a calm nervous system or a slow heart rate. When you start to feel your heart rate slowing (that's the feedback part), then you are on the right track. Focus on the thoughts that produce the desired results. You can do the same thing with muscle spasm and get feedback by placing your hand over the tight muscle.

Interactive Mindfulness for Parents and Premature Babies

With time, observation, and help from the nurses in the NICU, you can learn the cues that indicate your baby is stressed. (See chapter 8.) Positive interactions with your baby can help combat these negative effects. In the hospital, you have the added help of monitors to assess the effects of your efforts on your baby's heart rate, respiratory rate, and oxygen level.

The following are some positive ways to interact, reduce stress, and promote healthy organization of a premature baby's nervous system.

- **Touch** is soothing and can be very beneficial for development of the autonomic nervous system. In the NICU your baby can benefit greatly from kangaroo care (holding your baby skin to skin) and from being held during painful procedures. Initially the tubes and wires seem daunting, but your baby's nurse will help you. Within a few days you will become very adept at holding them with all the equipment.

- **Eye contact, smiling, and interacting** with your baby. Babies absorb every interaction with you—this is the model from which they learn. Unfortunately, because of physical challenges, many premature babies have fewer opportunities to interact, so it is important to use every opportunity when your baby is awake and receptive to this interaction.

- **Sucking a pacifier** is comforting for a premature baby and helps the developing nervous system form positive connections. Offer a pacifier at regular intervals and any time your baby appears stressed.

- **Working on good sleep patterns.** Rest and quiet allow the nervous system time to process input and is essential for the release of important hormones and chemicals that regulate all body systems.

Only one therapy seemed to help Victor's reflux—holding him upright against my chest. It's what we now call the *cuddle position*. On many nights his reflux and vomiting were so bad he could only sleep in this position, and so I held him and slept the best that I could, sitting in a recliner. This went on for more than a year. Many people are aghast at the thought, but holding him like that, feeling his muscles relax and his stomach settle, drinking in his warmth, was enormously comforting for both of us, and so the biofeedback went both ways.

The recliner has long been retired, but even now when Victor is bothered by his reflux, we will assume the cuddle position and I will think of nothing but trying to get our systems in sync. Gradually, I can feel his stiff body relax, the storm gurgling in his stomach will settle, and his hiccups fade to a memory. Once we are both fully relaxed, almost in a different plane of consciousness, he will whisper in my ear, "Tell me again, Momma, how we used to sleep in a chair." Inevitably, we are both sound asleep by the end of the first sentence.

PART FOUR

Making the System Work for You

16

Navigating Your Health Insurance

Health insurance is a complex system with bizarre regulations, and navigating it can often feel like playing a video game in a foreign language with rules that keep changing. However, understanding health insurance is essential, not only to minimize expenses, but to avoid delays in accessing the right medical care.

The Patient Protection and Affordable Care Act of 2010 (H.R. 3590) has changed health insurance, benefiting families with a premature baby. As of September 23, 2010, health insurance companies are prohibited from using pre-existing medical conditions to deny or limit coverage or to charge unrealistic rates for *children* in all new plans. Other positive changes for children starting September 2010 include the ability for parents to keep insuring their child on a family policy until their child reaches the age of 26 and the elimination of lifetime maximums (a limit on how much money the health plan will pay for medical care over the course of a lifetime).

The first step in navigating insurance is to understand your type of plan.

- **Group plans.** This is employer-sponsored health insurance. Almost 60 percent of Americans get their health insurance through their employers. The employer decides on the benefits and how much you pay for your health care. It is important to enroll your baby in your group plan within 30 days of birth or they may not be eligible for health insurance until open enrollment (generally held only once a year). In 2014, small businesses can band together to buy group insurance (this will help you get a better deal with the insurance company), making group insurance available to more Americans.

- **Individual plans.** This is health insurance purchased directly by an individual or a family. Before health care reform, people with pre-existing conditions or those at higher risk for medical conditions could be charged more or even denied insurance altogether. Individual plans are typically more expensive than group plans, but in 2014 subsidies will be available to help pay for individual insurance policies (depending on family income) if your employer does not provide health insurance.

- **Medicaid and the Children's Health Insurance Program (CHIP)** are government-funded health insurance programs for low-income people and people with certain disabilities. Many premature babies qualify for Medicaid or CHIP.

- **Medicare** is a federal health insurance plan for individuals over 65, for people under 65 who are on disability, and anyone on dialysis for kidney failure. A premature baby is unlikely to have Medicare.

- **High-risk pools** are state-sponsored health insurance plans for those who are denied individual coverage based on pre-existing medical conditions. In 2009, only 34 states had high-risk pools with some providing decent coverage at an affordable rate while others did not. A federal high-risk pool will start September 23, 2010, and will operate until 2014 when under the health reform law denial based on a pre-existing medical condition will no longer be allowed for anyone. Children no longer need high-risk pools as the health reform law exempts them from restrictions based on pre-existing conditions as of September 2010.

While both Oliver and Victor were still in the NICU, I received a hospital bill that left me physically ill. It was a $300 bill for Aidan's care. He has been charged a co-payment as if he were a full-term baby.

"I will sort this out," I told myself and called the billing department. Someone checked the wrong box. An unfortunate mistake, but I understood that things happen.

I was met with nothing but arguments. "He received some care," I was told. "Every baby does."

It took me a few minutes to compose myself. "You are mistaken," I replied. "He died." To revisit the trauma with an unsympathetic stranger was devastating.

She would not listen. "They would have given him care and medications before he died; you just didn't see it." She was completely deaf to my story.

Finally I explained that I was Dr. Gunter, an OB/GYN at the hospital, and that my son lived three minutes and only received a blanket. The answer: "You still owe us $300."

I was spewing tears of rage, violation, victimization, frustration, and pain. I couldn't believe it. Over the years I had heard stories of billing nightmares, but hadn't really understood that the system could be *so* inept.

I regained my composure and within the hour someone from hospital administration took care of the matter, but I never received an apology. I vowed to learn everything about insurance and medical billing, and now I know the system better than anyone. I wish I could say that was the end of our billing problems; however, being prepared has made the process easier.

Employer–Sponsored Group Health Insurance

There are three major types of group health insurance:

- **Health Maintenance Organization** (HMO). Health care is organized through your primary care provider (PCP); for your baby this may be a pediatrician, family doctor, or nurse practitioner. Referrals are required to see a specialist, and pre-authorization is required for some tests and procedures and all surgeries. Only services within an HMO's network of providers and hospitals are

covered. Out-of-network care is covered only in emergencies or
with special pre-approval.

- **Preferred provider organization** (PPO). A PPO plan provides
  more choices of providers and hospitals, and referrals are not
  needed to see a specialist, but there are more out-of-pocket expenses. A PPO plan has a preferred network of providers, but out-
  of-network care is allowed at a higher cost.
- **Point of service plan** (POS), a combination of an HMO and a
  PPO. In-network care runs like an HMO, and out-of-network care
  is available but more expensive.

When looking at health plans, most people think only about monthly
premiums, the amount it costs every month to keep the insurance. (Children's Medicaid and CHIP have no monthly premiums.) However, out-
of-pocket costs, the amount you actually pay to use your insurance, should
also be considered. Out-of-pocket costs include:

- **Co-payment,** a pre-determined fee paid at the time of care. Co-
  payments apply toward the deductible, but do not always count
  against the out-of-pocket maximum (see below). Co-payments
  can quickly add up when you use a lot of services. Insurances purchased on or after September 23, 2010, cannot charge co-payments
  for preventative care (often called well-baby or well-child visits)
  or vaccinations.
- **Deductible,** the amount of money that must be paid in out-of-
  pocket expenses each year before the insurance starts paying. It
  varies from plan to plan whether co-payments count towards
  the deductible. A premature baby's medical care in the first year
  will almost always surpass the deductible. There are also high-
  deductible health plans (HDHPs) with special features. An HDHP
  allows people to establish a special tax-exempt savings account to
  pay for expenses incurred before the deductible kicks in. An HDHP
  favors a family unlikely to have a lot of expenses, so most parents

with a premature baby are better off with a traditional deductible, and the lower the better.

- **Co-insurance,** the amount that you must pay for a service once the deductible is met. It's typically a percentage of the bill. If a bill is $1,000 but the deductible is $200 and the co-insurance is 80 percent, the amount that must be paid is $200 (the deductible) plus 20 percent of the difference between the bill and the deductible, in this case $160 (20 percent of $800). Co-insurance only applies to PPO plans and out-of-network care with a POS plan.

- **Out-of-pocket maximum,** a cap on expenses. Once the out-of-pocket maximum is reached for the year the insurance plan covers the co-insurance, although co-payments may still be required. A lower out-of-pocket maximum is preferable. Prescription drugs and mental health services may or may not count toward the out-of-pocket maximum. With a PPO plan there may be a separate out-of-pocket maximum for in-network and out-of-network care.

TABLE 1: Summary of Benefits Comparing HMO, POS, and PPO Plans

	HMO	POS	PPO
Providers and Hospitals	In-network only	Lowest cost in-network Higher cost out-of-network	Lowest cost in-network Higher cost out-of-network
Need for referral to see specialist	Yes	In-network: Yes Out-of-network: No	In-network: No Out-of-network: No
Pre-authorization for procedures and certain tests	Yes	Yes	Yes
Annual deductible	Varies by plan	In-network: Varies by plan Out-of-network: Yes	In-network: Usually Out-of-network: Yes and more expensive
Co-insurance	No	In-network: No Out-of-network: Yes	In-network: Yes Out-of-network: Yes and more expensive
Cost	$	$$	$$$

If you have a choice between plans look at the in-network doctors and hospitals. You need a health plan that allows you access to a pediatric hospital and a wide cadre of pediatric sub-specialists in the event they are needed. Also examine the types of services covered under the plan. Many premature babies need some or all of the following services, but they may be excluded or be limited with some health plans:

- **Physical, occupational, and speech therapy.** Premature babies may need weekly visits for their first year if not longer. Some health plans allow only 10 visits a year, and some plans don't cover physical or occupational therapy at all.
- **Durable medical equipment.** These are supplies like oxygen and feeding tubes. Plans may have a maximum allowable per year, a co-insurance, or a flat co-payment.
- **Mental health services.** Attention deficit disorder, autism, and behavioral problems are more common among premature babies. As children get older, help from psychologists, behavioral specialists, and psychiatrists can be invaluable

As medical expenses are likely to be higher, an HMO will almost always be less expensive for a family with a premature baby. A 2008 *Consumer Reports* survey on experience with health insurance indicates that people with HMOs pay less for premiums and have lower out-of-pocket expenses compared with those who have PPO plans. Billing errors were also much more common with PPO plans. (See Table 2 for a comparison of costs with four different insurance plans and the bill for one hospitalization). While a PPO plan does offer the freedom to see specialists without a referral, this survey indicates there was essentially no difference in the ability to access needed care—15 percent of HMO members and 14 percent of PPO members who were ill reported problems getting care.

PPOs also have a hidden charge called balanced billing. Co-insurance is based on what is called a customary and reasonable charge for a service (basically what an insurance plan is willing to pay for a service). If the hospital or doctor charges more than the PPO allows, the patient

TABLE 2: Out-of-Pocket Costs with Four Hypothetical Health Plans with a $50,000 NICU Bill

	HMO	POS in network	PPO 1	PPO 2
Deductible	None	$1,000	$500	$2,000
Co-payment/ co-insurance	$300 ($300 co-pay per hospital admission)	$1,000 ($250 co-pay per day, max allowable $1,000/ admission)	$9,900 (20 percent co-insurance, 49,500 x 0.20 = 9,900)	$14,400 (48,000 x 30 percent co-insurance = 14,400)
Bill	$300	$1,000	$10,400	$16,400
Out-of-pocket family maximum	None	None	$2,000	$12,000
Money owed	$300	$1,000	$2,000	$12,000

is responsible for the difference. For example, a hospital charges $7,000 for surgery but the insurance allows a customary and reasonable charge of $5,000. Using an insurance with a $1,000 deductible and an 80 percent co-insurance, the cost to the patient for this surgery rises from $1,800 (the $1,000 deductible *plus* $800 in co-insurance [20 percent of $4,000]) to $3,800 (deductible plus co-insurance *plus* the difference between $5,000 and $7,000), adding another $2,000 to the bill. Payments in excess of the "customary and reasonable" allowance do not always count toward the out-of-pocket maximum. Parents with a PPO should always ask up front about the cost of a procedure and check with their insurance company to see if it's considered in the customary and reasonable range. Not only will this prevent surprises, but it's often possible to negotiate the price with the doctor or hospital downward ahead of time. Balanced billing is not allowed with Medicaid and HMO plans.

Quality of care is also important. You can look up health plan performance at the NCQA (National Committee for Quality Assurance) web site, which publishes compliance with national standards and report cards on specific plans.

I took Oliver to an in-network urgent care clinic, presented both his HMO and his Medicaid card, and after his evaluation and chest X-ray learned that he had pneumonia and low oxygen. We were transferred by ambulance to our in-network hospital, where he was hospitalized for eight days.

A month or so later I receive a bill for the X-ray taken at the urgent care clinic. My HMO denied it, as the X-ray facility was actually part of a non-network hospital. "No problem," I thought. "This is a simple error of not submitting the X-ray as urgent/emergent, and if I can't correct that problem, we have the Medicaid as backup."

I called the non-network hospital, explained that the bill should be coded as urgent or emergent, and asked that they re-submit. I also indicated Oliver had Medicaid, so we shouldn't really be getting billed anyway. I faxed a follow-up letter, to be on the safe side.

The next month another bill arrived for the same chest X-ray. I called my insurance, and much to my surprise I found that the bill had never been re-submitted.

So I called and sent another follow-up letter. Over the next four months, this same scenario repeated itself over and over. I could not make any "billing specialist" understand the difference between a routine and urgent X-ray or make them re-submit the bill correctly to my HMO or Medicaid. They only wanted to charge me.

I was threatened with collections. I called Medicaid to confirm that Oliver's coverage was active at the time of the X-ray and called the State Attorney General's office in Colorado to confirm the Colorado Medicaid law. I sent a letter to the non-network hospital detailing all that information, even quoting the Colorado statute enacted to supposedly protect people from this kind of predatory activity.

We were sent to collections.

I contacted the collections agency. They didn't care about the billing error and when it came to Oliver's Medicaid, the answer was, "Prove it."

I called Medicaid and got a Medspan report, a legal document proving Medicaid coverage. I faxed it and also sent it registered. I then sent a letter to the CEO of the non-network hospital, because CEOs hate to be bothered by angry patients. To ensure he received the letter, I faxed it to his personal fax and mailed it certified. To make sure my letter really caught his attention, I indicated that I was also sending it to a newspaper, the Colorado office of Medicaid Fraud, the Colorado Insurance Commissioner, the Attorney General, and a TV station. I received a call within 24 hours indicating the bill would be pulled from collections. I never received an apology.

But it gets worse. When I spoke to Medicaid about the Medpsan, they kindly reviewed the charges. There was a very long pause before the woman on the other end of the phone spoke. "It's interesting that you have been billed," she said, "because Medicaid paid that claim back in November 2005." When the mess was finally untangled, the billing department at the non-network hospital had generated two chest X-ray bills instead of one. My HMO had denied both claims, not only because they were billed as non-urgent, but also because two claims for identical procedures on the same day is an automatic denial. Instead of reviewing their paperwork for errors and then re-submitting to my HMO, which would have paid a correct bill, the hospital took the easy road and billed the taxpayers for two chest X-rays. Medicaid paid one and of course denied the obvious error. This yearlong ordeal was for a duplicate X-ray that had never even existed.

Government-Funded Plans

Medicaid and the Children's Health Insurance Program (SCHIP) provide health insurance for millions of children in the United States. A premature baby may qualify for regular Medicaid based on a family income at or below 133 percent of the Federal Poverty Level (FPL). The actual dollar amount depends on the number of family members in the household and changes every year. Some states have less restrictive eligibility requirements to include more children. For example, in 2009 California allowed a family income of 200 percent of the FPL for Medicaid eligibility.

In 39 states many premature children can qualify for Medicaid at birth, *regardless of parental income*, based on their Social Security Income (SSI) eligibility (see chapter 18). Medical conditions that qualify a premature baby for SSI without considering their parent's income include low birth weight or a major birth defect that would be life threatening without immediate surgery, such as a heart defect. The following states have more restrictive criteria for Medicaid than SSI eligibility: Connecticut, Hawaii, Illinois, Indiana, Minnesota, Missouri, New Hampshire North Dakota, Ohio, Oklahoma, and Virginia.

Ask a social worker to help you start the Medicaid paperwork while your baby is in the hospital. You don't have to be a U.S. citizen, or even a legal immigrant, for your baby to get Medicaid.

CHIP is a state-run health insurance for children and has less restrictive income requirements than Medicaid. Like Medicaid, income requirements vary from state to state. For example, in 2009 in North Dakota the family income requirement for CHIP was 150 percent of FPL, and in New Jersey it was 350 percent. CHIP is typically less inclusive than Medicaid, meaning there are fewer covered services or you have a more limited network of providers. CHIP may become available to more children under the health care reform act of 2010.

Children who are eligible for regular Medicaid typically have no co-payments, so there are very few out-of-pocket expenses. The only time a children's Medicaid recipient can be billed is if the provider/hospital informs the parents beforehand in writing that the service in not a covered benefit *and* you sign a specific waiver agreeing. CHIP has co-payments—they vary from state to state but typically range from $1 to $5. Additional billing is also not allowed under CHIP. When doctors or hospitals accept Medicaid or CHIP, they must accept what the state is willing to pay them.

There is a lot of variation among the states regarding benefits covered by Medicaid and CHIP and rules often change. Read everything that comes in the mail from your Medicaid office. Medicaid offices typically also have very comprehensive Web sites.

If your baby's Medicaid is based on SSI eligibility (birth weight or birth defects), she will be reassessed at one year of age. The state Medicaid offices are often behind on these assessments, so the first contact may be several months after your baby's first birthday. In some cases a health care professional, typically a doctor or physical therapist, does an evaluation and recommends for or against further coverage. Sometimes there is no assessment and simply an automatic termination of benefits. If Medicaid is terminated at one year, you can appeal the decision. The process varies from state to state.

Many Medicaid and CHIP plans are administered by HMOs, with the same doctors and hospitals as employer-sponsored insurance, although the government decides on the covered services. Enrollment in an HMO may be mandatory, and in this case it's important for you to pick your child's primary care doctor, otherwise one will be assigned. Like any HMO, non-emergency care outside of the Medicaid/CHIP network may not be covered.

Dealing with Two Insurances

Some families are fortunate enough to have two insurances. While this expands benefits, extra paperwork and specific rules are involved, increasing the risk of billing errors. There are two scenarios where this can happen:

- **Group insurance and Medicaid.** This happens when you have health insurance through work and your baby has Medicaid based on birth weight. Medicaid is always the insurance of last resort, so your group insurance is billed first. However, Medicaid exempts you from co-payments and co-insurance for covered benefits.
- **Two different group insurances.** This may happen when both parents are working. If the insurance is free or at a very low rate, it makes sense to enroll in both plans. The rule designating the primary insurance for the children is odd: The parent whose birthday falls earlier in the calendar year is designated as having the primary insurance (age, or birth year, doesn't matter). All the rules of the first insurance must be followed before the second insurance can be billed. For example, if your first plan is an HMO and the second plan is a PPO, before going to a doctor in the PPO, you need a denial letter from the HMO, because going out of network is not a covered benefit under your HMO.

The Nuances of Working a Health Plan

Failure to follow health plan rules can lead to delays in care, mountains of paperwork, and unnecessary expenses. The most important things to keep in mind are:

- **The need for pre-authorization.** This is advance permission for certain procedures (like surgery), certain tests (such as an MRI), and some medications. Pre-authorization is not a guarantee that your insurance company will pay; however, without pre-authorization the insurance company has no obligation to pay. Pre-authorization is not required in emergency situations or for procedures, tests, or medications that take place during a hospital stay. To avoid delays and surprise bills, always ask if pre-authorization is required—call your insurance carrier, because your provider may not be up-to-date on health plan specifics. If you need pre-authorization, call your insurance to be sure the doctor or hospital submitted the paperwork *and* get the pre-authorization number for your own records. When you register for the procedure or test, double check with the staff to make sure they have the correct pre-authorization number. *One of the biggest traps for pre-authorization is when a doctor suggests an unplanned procedure at an office visit.* Yes, it is easier to just go ahead and do it, but the insurance company will not authorize a procedure after the fact. It's best to ask the doctor to obtain the pre-authorization first, even if that means waiting in the office or rescheduling for another day.
- **The difference between emergency room visits and urgent care.** Many urgent and after-hours problems can be handled in an urgent care clinic. Urgent care visits have the same co-payment as an office visit, much lower than the co-payment for an emergency room visit (which is often $100 or higher). Most urgent care clinics have access to X-rays, can perform some tests, and can look after many problems that are too acute for a regular doctor's office. An

urgent care clinic cannot handle true emergencies. Urgent care clinics are also convenient, because the wait times are typically shorter.

- **If your baby is admitted to the hospital within 24 hours of an emergency room (ER) visit, the ER co-pay is typically waived.** Keep your receipts. If you paid your ER co-payment at the time, make sure that amount is credited toward your final bill. If you didn't pay the ER co-payment, make sure you are not billed for it.

- **Make sure every provider is on your plan.** Even though you may be using an in-network hospital, not every provider is necessarily in your network. It's an outrage that a parent can receive pre-authorized care at an in-network hospital only to be shocked with a bill from an out-of-network provider. It's hard to ask everyone if they're on a specific health plan, but a good rule of thumb is to go by the name badge. If the in-network facility name is not on the hospital name tag, chances are higher that person may be an out-of-network provider. Speak up and insist on in-network personnel.

- **Negotiate bills in advance.** Parents with a co-insurance (PPO plan) and even parents who are paying entirely out of pocket can discuss payment options with the hospital financial counselor. A lower price or an interest-free payment plan (a far better option than a credit card) can often be negotiated.

Specialist Referrals

To see a specialist in an HMO, in-network POS, and most Medicaid plans, you need a referral. The billing staff from your primary care provider's office will contact the insurance company for the referral. Once the appointment is made, the specialist's staff should double check for the referral. Just as with pre-authorization, do not assume everything is in place. Contact your insurance company for the referral number and bring it to the appointment. It's incredibly frustrating to show up at the specialist's office, expectations high, only to be turned away because of lack of a referral or to be required to pay for the services without knowing if you'll be reimbursed.

Deconstructing Medical Bills

Billing errors are common. To prevent or mitigate problems, you must:

- **Understand your plan benefits** so you know what is covered and what is out of pocket.
- **Keep records** of doctors' names, procedures, and therapies. Billing errors frequently include charges for services that were never rendered.
- **Know how to read and interpret a medical bill.** A doctor's office has one bill. If your baby was in the hospital, there will be two bills, one from the hospital and one from the doctors. The statements will indicate what portion of the bill is your responsibility as well as what has been billed to your insurance. If your baby has Medicaid, you should not owe anything. If you have an HMO and the service was pre-approved, then you should only have your co-payment, which goes to the hospital. (If you have an HMO, you don't pay a co-payment for the doctor's services in the hospital.) PPO bills are the most confusing, as there are co-payments, deductibles, and co-insurances. What you have to pay with a PPO is usually a percentage of the actual cost, so it's essential to scour the bill for errors.
- **Read the explanation of benefits.** This describes the services performed and the associated charges. If the insurance company is denying a claim, there will be an explanation. Check the explanation of benefits against your records for accuracy. Call immediately if you notice discrepancies.

Never ignore a billing error. Failure to pay, even if the bill is incorrect, can lead to referral to a collection agency. Appeal every incorrect bill (doctor's office or hospital) in writing. State specifically that you dispute the bill and why. The two biggest errors are:

- **Denial of services,** meaning the insurance company rejects the entire claim. Reasons for denial are incorrectly submitted paperwork, failure to obtain pre-authorization, not a covered benefit, or out-of-network care (for an HMO only). Incorrectly submitted paperwork can be re-submitted if done in a timely manner. However, there is generally no way around denials for out-of-network care for non-emergency services and failure to obtain pre-authorization.
- **Charges for services or procedure that never happened.** Approximately 80 percent of medical bills contain this kind of error. Ask for an itemized bill. Common errors include the number of days in the hospital or being billed for a service that never took place.

17

<hr />

Prescription Drugs

Most people with employer-sponsored insurance have prescription medication coverage. However, even then many people have problems getting the medication they need due to complex rules and out-of-pocket expenses. Many parents pay more than they should for medications, or worse, go without. Not surprisingly, families with no health insurance have the hardest time.

Every health plan has a formulary, which is a list of preferred medications. Formularies are divided into tiers that separate preferred drugs from non-preferred medications (see Figure 10) by price. Preferred medications have the lowest co-payments to encourage use. Formulary drugs are also divided into generic and brand name. Some plans allow non-formulary drugs at a higher cost, while others don't cover non-formulary drugs at all.

The out-of-pocket expenses for prescription medications are typically based on a 30-day supply. Co-payments are usually fixed amounts; however, some plans have co-insurance, which is a percentage of the cost of the drug. Brand-name drugs are expensive, so with co-insurance, out-of-pocket costs can quickly escalate. With most plans, money paid on prescription drugs contributes to the deductible, but some insurance plans have separate deductibles and out-of-pocket maximums for medications.

Regular Medicaid and CHIP have two tiers: formulary and non-formulary. Only formulary drugs are covered, and the formularies vary

FIGURE 10: Breakdown of Prescription Medication Formulary

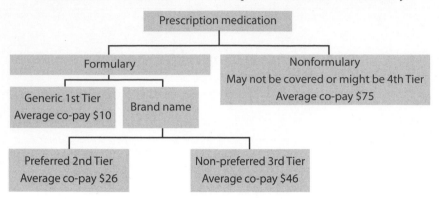

from state to state. There may be a low co-payment (generally from $1 to $5 for a 30-day supply) or no co-payment at all.

What exactly is a generic medication? Medications have two names, a generic and a brand name. The generic name refers to the chemical name of the drug, and the brand name is what the company has named it. For example, *Tylenol* is a brand name and *acetaminophen* is the generic name. A generic drug has the same active ingredient(s), meaning the part of the drug that actually works, but the inactive ingredients, or fillers, may vary.

The company that does the original research makes brand-name drugs. Once the FDA approves a brand-name drug, the patent is protected for 10 years. After this time is up, other companies are free to produce the drug, but a generic manufacturer has to first prove to the FDA that its drug is equivalent to the original brand-name version.

A good analogy is the "no-name brand" concept at the grocery store. When thinking of ketchup, most people think of Heinz. The primary ingredients that make ketchup are tomatoes, vinegar, and sugar; however, there may be minor variations in spices and additives between brands. Nonetheless, they are all ketchup.

There are companies that specifically make generics, but the original brand-name company often makes its own generics. (The companies have all the equipment, so a generic is another way to continue profiting from the drug.) The manufacturer of every generic is listed in an FDA publication called the Orange Book, found online. (Go to www. preemieprimer.com for links.)

For most drugs, there's no practical difference between generic and brand name. If a problem or a safety concern exists with the generic, it typically exists for the brand name as well. Switching from brand name to a generic (when one becomes available) and between different generic manufacturers is common practice, because there is competition, and one manufacturer may offer your pharmacy a better price. For most medical conditions, this kind of switching will be imperceptible. However, there is some evidence that problems can occur with constant switching of medications for epilepsy, so parents who have children on anti-seizure medication should be especially vigilant about these switches, and any change in seizure activity should be reported to the prescribing doctor. This is a case in which appealing for the brand-name version might be advisable in order to avoid the shell game of rotating generics.

Other important information about generic drugs:

- **There are no studies comparing brand-name drugs head-to-head with their generic competitors.** There is no medical reason not to try a generic if available.
- **Using generics saves billions of dollars every year** in health care costs that would otherwise be transferred back to you in the form of increased premiums, out-of-pocket expenses, or both.
- **Even if a prescription is for a brand-name drug, if a generic is available, the insurance company will insist on the generic** unless the provider writes "no substitution" on the prescription. Even then, insisting on a brand name when a generic is available is a common reason for denial.
- **Sometimes there is no generic for a particular medication, so the insurance company will try to substitute a similar medication that has a generic.** This is not the same as switching from a brand name to a generic; this is like switching from ketchup to tomato sauce. It is a *change* in the prescription. It's important to

check with the doctor before accepting such a switch, even if it means calling the doctor's office from the pharmacy.

Medication costs can quickly add up, even with generics, and some babies may be on two or three medications every month in addition to one or two rounds of antibiotics or other medications throughout the year. Asking for generics, if available, is one way to keep costs down. Other cost-saving tips include:

- **Asking for the largest prescription your insurance will allow.** Some health plans require a new co-payment/co-insurance for every 30-day supply, but others allow a 90-day supply.
- **Sign up for mail order** if available, as most insurances allow a 90-day supply for the cost of one or two 30-day co-payments, saving you 30 percent or more on drug costs a year. The insurance company pays the shipping, so there is no cost for gas or parking. Call at least 10 days in advance for mail-order refills to allow ample time for delivery.
- **If your generic co-payment is greater than $5, the medication may be cheaper to purchase outside of the health plan.** A 30-day supply of many generics is available at many Target and Wal-Mart stores for $4.
- **Use your cafeteria plan if one is available.** A cafeteria plan is an employer-sponsored benefit that allows you to put pre-tax dollars aside to pay for medical expenses such as prescription and non-prescription medications (as well as co-payments and co-insurance). You must provide receipts to get reimbursed.

Pre-authorizations, Denials, and Appeals

Issues getting generic medications are rare; however, many brand-name drugs require pre-authorization. This means that someone from the doctor's office (doctor or nurse) has to explain (either over the phone or in writing) to the insurance carrier why the medication is needed. Sometimes it's just a formality, but other times it's a very arduous process. Common reasons for pre-authorization:

- **The drug is not the preferred formulary choice or is non-formulary.**
- **The medication is prescribed for an off-label indication.** This means the drug is being prescribed outside of the use it was approved for by the FDA. This is common practice for babies less than one year old, as studies are almost never performed on children this young.

It's very aggravating to get to the pharmacy and find out a medication needs pre-authorization. Chances are the prescribing provider did not know, as most accept more than 10 insurance plans and the formulary for each plan is constantly changing.

If the medication is denied, the options are to go without the drug, pay out of pocket, ask your doctor to prescribe a formulary alternative, or launch an appeal. An appeal is generally worthwhile, as it costs nothing (except time and emotional energy).

The insurance company will mail a letter within a few days detailing the reasons for the denial and the necessary steps for appeal. Pay attention to time limits. For a successful appeal, you must prove why that specific medication is needed. Helpful information to provide:

- **Details of the medical condition.**
- **Medical evidence to support the use of this medication for the specific medical condition.** You may need to include reference to at least one medical study (two is better) as well as a letter detailing why the medication is needed. Guidelines supporting the use of the medication from the American Academy of Pediatrics or another medical organization are also helpful. Ask your doctor to direct you to the right study or these published guidelines. Go to www.preemieprimer.com to download a template for an appeal letter.

- Proof that the cheaper generic and preferred brand-name formulary medications have been tried and failed.
- Proof that the formulary drug cannot be used because of an allergy, an adverse reaction, or other health reasons.
- Proof that the FDA-approved medications have been tried and failed or that there is no FDA-approved medication for this condition.

If a non-formulary medication is denied and your health plan doesn't cover non-formulary drugs, an appeal is unlikely to be successful, although it's always worth a try if there is simply no formulary alternative. A useful line to consider including in an appeal letter is this: "As there are no formulary-approved medications, it appears that you are in effect excluding all persons with this medical condition from therapy." The appeal letter should be copied to your state insurance commissioner and the benefits person for your employer if you have group insurance. You can also file a formal complaint with the state insurance commissioner; however, if you have self-funded health insurance (meaning your employer has devoted funds to cover all the health plan expenses and the insurance company is simply doing the administrative aspect), your appeal against your insurance carrier is exempt from review by the state insurance commissioner.

Special Medication Issues

Injectables

Injectable medications are typically in their own medication class because of their expense. They almost always require pre-authorization. The injectable medication most parents will encounter is *Synagis*, a vaccine that protects against respiratory syncytial virus (RSV). *Synagis* is approximately $900 per injection, and many premature babies will need up to five injections to get through their first winter. The pre-authorization should be relatively straightforward, as prematurity is the prime indication; however, call a few days after the paperwork has been submitted to proactively deal with any problems. The American Academy of Pediatrics has published guidelines for the use of *Syngis* and should be referenced in any appeal process (available at www.preemieprimer.com).

Compounding

For many children, the lowest-strength pill made contains too much drug. To get the right dose, the medication must be specially mixed or compounded by a pharmacist. Most chain pharmacies, like Target and Walgreens, don't do compounding. It's always best to call to see if a pharmacy compounds before taking the prescription in.

Unfortunately, insurance issues are common. Many plans consider compounded medications to be non-formulary, and sometimes they are not covered at all. Chances are better that the compounded medication will be covered if the actual drug to be compounded is on the formulary. Many times, compounded prescriptions will be denied; however, because the amount of drug to be used is actually very small, the cost of the drug may be less than you think.

People often ask if I get angry about the price of prescription medications. The fact that I routinely answer no surprises a lot of people.

My issue is not with the pharmaceutical companies (affectionately known as Big Pharma)—for the most part, they're following the rules that our government allows.

In 2008, 12 pharmaceutical executives were each paid $12 million or more in salary. Many use a company jet or helicopter. Drug companies spend more than $4 billion a year advertising their medications directly to consumers. Tens of millions of dollars, and in some cases more than $200 million, can be spent advertising *just one drug* over the course of just one year. Pharmaceutical companies also spend more than $100 million a year on Washington lobbyists to secure their investments. They are getting what they paid for and they are not breaking any laws. So who is *really* at fault?

18

<hr/>

Government and Other
Assistance Programs

There are many government and private programs that can provide assistance for you and your baby. With federal programs, the rules are the same no matter where you live in the United States. However, there are also many state, county, and school district services as well as private programs, so what is available where you live and how you can access it can vary significantly. One rule that applies to every service is *keep copies of everything so you have a paper trail.* Write down the date you mailed any paperwork on your copy, or send it with delivery confirmation. If you fax, keep the proof of delivery. Keep a binder with all your communication (copies of letters and faxes) and log every phone call (date and time), what was said, and who said it.

Supplemental Security Income or SSI

Social Security is a financial assistance program. Any money received by your child because of a disability is called Supplemental Security Income (SSI).

Eligibility involves the nature of the disability as well as the income and resources of family members living at home. However, *many premature babies who are hospitalized are eligible for SSI based on birth weight regardless of their family's financial situation.* (See Table 1.) There are also

TABLE 1: Birth Weight Criteria for SSI (No Financial Eligibility Requirements)

Gestational Age at Birth	Birth Weight
Any	< 1,200 g (2 lbs, 2 oz)
33 weeks	1,350 g (2 lbs, 15 oz) or less
34 weeks	1,500 g (3 lbs, 5 oz) or less
35 weeks	1,700 g (3 lbs, 12 oz) or less
36 weeks	1,875 g (4 lbs, 2 oz) or less

specific medical conditions that qualify a baby for SSI regardless of family income. Your NICU social worker should have the forms, but you can also find them online at www.SSI.gov. You can also call the 800 number to register your baby, but your child may not yet have a Social Security number, which increases the chance for error with phone applications. Applying for SSI is very important, because in 39 states having SSI automatically qualifies your baby for Medicaid, which will lower your health care expenses considerably.

While your baby is hospitalized you will receive $30 a month from SSI (retroactive to the date you filed), but it takes four to six weeks for the checks to start showing up. The money should be spent toward the care of your child. In the hospital, that can include gas, parking, and meals, and after discharge, SSI can be used for medical expenses or bottles, food, clothes, and diapers. You can also put the money in a bank account for your baby.

SSI rules are very specific. (See Figure 11.) When your baby is discharged and brought home, you must report her change of address, and your income now becomes a factor in maintaining eligibility. You can call the 800 number or get the paperwork online. To remain eligible, your baby's disability must be severe, she must be expected to remain disabled at least 12 months, and the household resources must be less than $3,000. (Resources are anything that could be sold for cash, except your house.) Social Security is supposed to reassess your baby's eligibility before she is six months old, but they are frequently behind schedule.

FIGURE 11: SSI flowchart

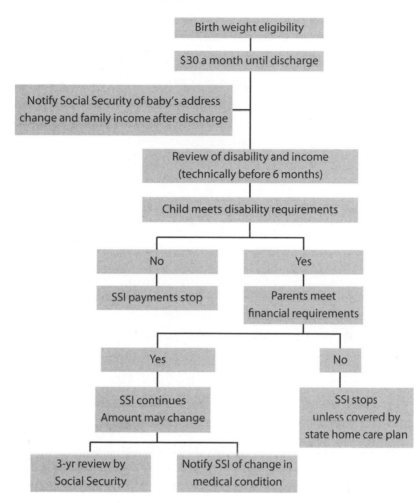

If you suspect that you don't meet the financial eligibility but the checks keep coming for more than a few months after you get home, send a letter with return receipt to your local Social Security office explaining the issue. *Social Security considers it your responsibility to contact them if you suspect an overpayment.* You will have to repay an overpayment unless you can prove it was the fault of Social Security *and* that you spent the money on your disabled child *and* that repayment would be a hardship.

If your baby remains eligible for SSI, the payments will depend on your monthly household income, how many children live at home, and where you live. (Some states provide a supplement to the federal payment.) The maximum federal payment in 2009 was $674 a month. (This changes every year.) You must report any change in household income by mail or fax before the 10th of every month. If Social Security deems your income to be too high, the amount of the check will be reduced or the payment suspended for that month. If you go 12 months with income that is too high, SSI will be terminated.

Your baby's eligibility for SSI will be reassessed in three years, but you must notify Social Security beforehand if your baby's health improves. If you have SSI, even for a few months, read the document *What You Need to Know When You Get Supplemental Security Income (SSI)* (available at www.preemieprimer.com).

If you're financially eligible but SSI does not consider your baby severely disabled, you may appeal. Talk to your baby's doctors and therapists for their opinions. You can do the appeal yourself, but there are tight deadlines and specific ways you must appeal, so many people hire a disability attorney. You do not have to pay up front—the attorney can charge up to 25 percent of any back payments as a fee (up to a certain amount).

Women, Infants, and Children (WIC)

WIC is a program that provides assistance for mothers who are breast-feeding or have children under the age of five, have low to medium incomes, and are at high risk for nutritional challenges. Checks or vouchers for nutritious food are provided, but some agencies distribute food packages. Formula may also be available. If your doctor recommends a special formula, you may be able to get it through WIC. Services also include education about nutrition, help finding health care, and liaison with other community resources.

Your family income must be below 185 percent of the Federal Poverty Level (FPL) to quality. The actual dollar amount changes every year, so check with a social worker online to see if you qualify. In 2009 a family of four could qualify for WIC with an annual income of $40,793 or less.

If you did not apply for WIC during your pregnancy, apply while your baby is in the hospital. Ask a social worker for help with the application. Applying as early as possible is important, because often there are waiting lists. Those with the greatest medical need, such as a premature baby, are given priority; however, funds are limited and you may have to wait for another family to graduate before you can start.

Government Early Intervention Services

According to Part C of the Individuals with Disabilities Education Act (IDEA), infants and toddlers with disabilities are eligible to receive services, regardless of their parent's income, to help them reach their full potential. The idea is that earlier intervention provides more benefit. Every state *must* provide these services. The money comes from Medicaid (federal government), state and local governments, the Department of Education, grants, and private fundraising.

A wide range of services may be available, including assessments and therapy (physical, occupational, and speech) and liaisons with other programs. Other services might include behavior programs, assistance with transportation, and medical equipment. Funding varies dramatically, even from county to county, so available services vary significantly by region.

To qualify for services, you must live in the service area and have a child under the age of three with a developmental delay. Children older than three may also be eligible if they have a disabling condition such as cerebral palsy, an intellectual disability, epilepsy, or autism.

Registration is required. Your social worker can help, and in some counties a representative from the program makes regular trips to the NICU to help parents enroll. Babies are assigned a case manager who will visit the home shortly after discharge. Case managers facilitate a Family Individual Program Plan (FIPP), which includes developmental goals and the services your baby needs to meet those goals. A medical assessment (by a doctor or one or more therapists) may be needed to help determine services.

School District

If your child has delays in key areas important for scholastic performance, particularly speech, fine motor skills, and social behavior, she may be eligible for services through your school district when she turns three. These services are part of an Individualized Educational Program, or IEP. To find out whether your child may be eligible, familiarize yourself with your state's standards for grade-level learning objectives. (This information is available online, or you can ask the district to mail it to you.)

Your IDEA case manager should arrange the meeting, but you can also request an assessment before or after your child starts attending school. Submit a letter specifically asking for an IEP evaluation—detail problems that you feel will affect (or is already affecting) your child's ability to learn and/or interact in a school setting. Include a letter of support from your child's doctors and therapists documenting specific areas of concern. Ask for a written response within 30 days.

The first step toward an IEP is a meeting with a school administrator. Other attendees may include a special education teacher, an occupation or speech therapist, and, if your child is already in school, one or more of her teachers. At this meeting you will present your concerns and provide medical records that describe delays and supporting letters from medical professionals. Provide specific examples of why you think your child is behind in speech, language, fine motor skills, or social behavior in comparison to the developmental milestones (if she is three to five years old) or grade-level standards (if she is already in school). This is also a good time to discuss any physical accommodations your child may need. For example, a child with significant visual impairment from retinopathy or prematurity may need visual aids and other classroom accommodations.

At this first meeting, the school district should document your concerns, assess your child's educational needs, and arrange standardized

I first met with the school district when Oliver and Victor turned three. Despite Oliver's speech being largely unintelligible and Victor still suffering from some significant sensory integration issues (he was unable to drink without help), I was told they were not as delayed as some of the other children who were receiving services. In reply, the phrase I found most helpful was, "I am not talking about other children, I am talking about Oliver and Victor." I was also prepared to discuss how Victor's inability to eat would affect his ability to go to school, as elementary children are expected to stay on campus during meals. I provided letters from their pediatrician and occupational therapist documenting their deficits.

They were enrolled in a special education preschool class and made incredible progress. One of the teachers decided Victor would be drinking unassisted from a cup before the year was over. I was doubtful, because spilling was a given due to his tremor, and he couldn't handle the sensation of being wet. He also hated the feel of the cup on his lips. Many meals resulted in screaming, arm flapping, and tears on everyone's part. It took her six months of dedicated work, but she managed.

Getting services requires sitting down to write a list of your child's deficits, and it's hard. Even now we are involved in a constant stream of discussion with the school about how best to help the boys. When I think I can't do it anymore, I think about Victor drinking from a cup, give myself a week or more, and then double my efforts.

assessments. If they adopt a "let's wait and see" attitude or indicate that your child does not qualify for services, be firm but polite and refer back to specific areas where you feel your child is behind. This is where letters from doctors and medical records from your pediatrician can be helpful.

You will meet again to discuss the results of assessments and arrange services if your child qualifies. There will be a document for you to sign, but *never sign anything you have not had time to read or do not agree with 100 percent*. You want to be able to digest the recommendations, cross out anything you disagree with, or write in addenda if needed.

If your child qualifies for an IEP, the school district can provide services such as speech therapy, occupational therapy, and behavioral therapy. This may include special classes, small group resources, classroom aids, or individual work with a therapist or special education teacher. If your child does not qualify for an IEP but there are recognized concerns, your school may come up with a "soft plan," not a formal IEP but some extra support and services.

There will be ongoing IEP meetings in which you will discuss your child's progress and the need for continuing services. Don't accept statements such as "Mary is doing better." Ask for specific examples of improvement, for example, "Mary's vocabulary has increased from 50 to 200 words."

Children with mild delays often fall through the cracks. Most schools want to help your child and would provide services if they could; however, budgets are tight. Talk with other parents who have successfully navigated the system *at your school* and gather concrete information and examples to illustrate your concerns. A private assessment with an occupational or speech therapist, developmental psychologist, or behavior specialist may also help.

It's emotionally draining when you think your child deserves services and the school district disagrees. Try to remain calm. Rehearsing can really pay off, so try writing what you want to say on cue cards. If tensions arise and the meeting becomes adversarial, it will only be counterproductive. Remember the goal: helping your child. If you feel your child is eligible for services and you're not getting what you need, you can also engage the services of a disability attorney.

Special Interest Groups

It's easy to find advocacy groups for practically every medical condition online, from autism to cerebral palsy. Advocacy groups can provide both support and practical advice. These parents understand what you're going through. The other irreplaceable service is inside information: services and treatments you may not have heard about and tricks on working the system. Try to connect with people who have children who are a few years older than yours. Most are only too willing to share their insight.

Steer clear of anyone who advocates only one or two therapies and promises cures. If it sounds too good to be true, it *is* too good to be true. Although there are excellent blogs with a wealth of valuable information, some people report inaccurate information, sometimes in good faith and sometimes with financial or political agendas. The Internet is a great place to get ideas and do research, but know your source and have a critical eye for every piece of information, whether it comes from a doctor or the Internet.

We learned about a great service at the most unlikely of places: a dinner party. When the boys were 18 months we had our first night out with friends. The conversation eventually turned to the boys and I spoke about our developmental concerns, which were more apparent each day.

A guest, whom we had never met, told us about the Rise School, a preschool for both special needs and regular track children. It was a protective environment with a 1:4 teacher-to-student ratio, physical and occupational therapy, and a developmental curriculum. It sounded like a dream.

The next day I called. It was everything we were told and more. And they had two openings! I signed them up on the spot. The boys attended the school for just one year, but their improvements were amazing.

The Rise School was the most nurturing and medically and developmentally appropriate program for our boys, and if we had never gone out to dinner that night we might never have known.

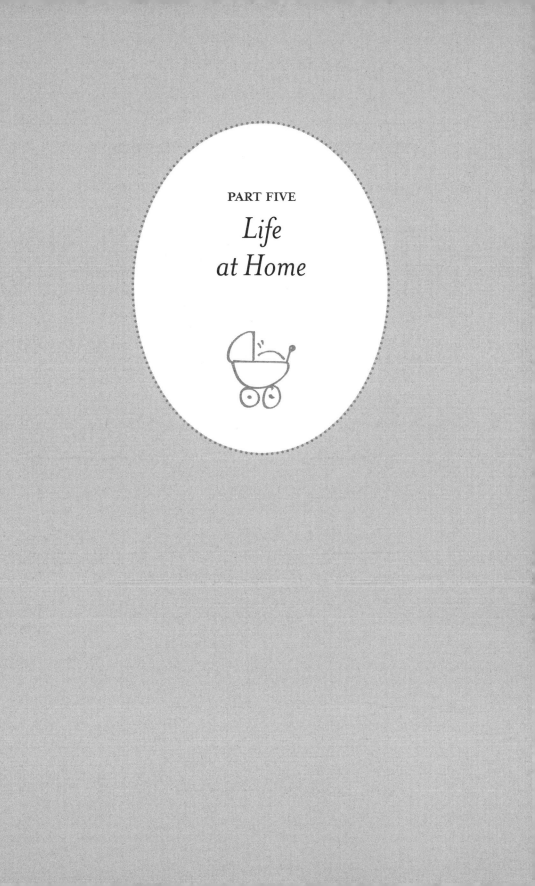

PART FIVE

*Life
at Home*

19

*Going
Home*

It may be hard to believe that your baby can manage without recording every breath and heartbeat, but eventually that time will come. It's impossible to predict when your baby will be discharged. There are no specific age or weight criteria; instead, the ability to go home is based on several milestones:

- **Maintaining a body temperature of 36.5° C (97.7° F)** in a crib at room temperature. (An extra blanket is acceptable.) This is unlikely before a weight of 1,800 g (4 lbs).
- **Appropriate weight gain.**
- **Absence of bradycardia episodes** (heart rate less than 80 beats/minute for five seconds) for several days.
- **Ability to maintain sufficient oxygen levels.** Supplemental oxygen to maintain these levels is fine as long as it will be used at home.
- **Passing a room air challenge test** if going home on oxygen. This is the ability to maintain an oxygen saturation of at least 80 percent without bradycardia for 40 minutes off oxygen. The purpose is to find out what would happen if the oxygen were to accidentally dislodge at home.
- **Being comfortable with feeding, medications, and equipment.**

Many NICUs have parent overnight rooms where you can spend a day or two caring for your baby with the doctors, nurses, and respiratory therapists literally just down the hall. This can increase your comfort level and may help ease the transition home.

Equipment Considerations

Some babies need special equipment at home. This is also called **durable medical equipment (DME).** The most common pieces of equipment are oxygen, feeding tubes, and an apnea monitor. While daunting at first, they're not difficult to master—most people use more complex and dangerous devices every day, such a gas stove or a car.

DME comes from a medical supply company and requires a prescription. Your baby's nurse or a social worker will help arrange the first delivery. They will know if you need equipment that day (such as oxygen or a monitor) or if it can wait a day or two. The hospital will provide you

I was more than apprehensive about changing the first oxygen tank at home. It's a lot different when you're in the hospital and the RT is standing over your shoulder. At home all I could think was that I was going to mess it up and the tank would either blow up, killing us all, or malfunction and deprive Oliver of oxygen.

Tony stepped in and switched the regulator to a different tank as if he had done it a thousand times! I was amazed. Yes, I am the medical person, but he understands everything mechanical.

Being at home with Oliver that first day, I felt completely unprepared. The checklist of things to do was just too long, never mind the feeling that I might somehow hurt Oliver by doing something wrong *and* the stress of Victor still being in the hospital. Having someone else there was invaluable. It took me a week to feel comfortable changing the tanks. I still had visions of complete and utter disaster, but before long I was changing the regulators as expertly as if I had been doing it my whole life.

with enough supplies until that first delivery. Once you get home, you'll need to arrange a delivery schedule.

Nasogastric Tube

Going home with a nasogastric tube (NG tube) is not uncommon. It can take weeks, or even longer, for some babies to learn to eat. As long as your baby is gaining weight, using an NG tube should not delay discharge. Being at home is less stressful, which may help speed up the process of learning to eat. To manage an NG tube at home, you must be able to do the following:

- Administer the feeds.
- Remove and replace the NG tube.
- Know how to care for the skin in and around the nose to prevent injury from the tube and the tape.

Home Oxygen

At home, oxygen for premature babies is supplied in pressurized tanks with a regulator that controls the flow of oxygen. The regulator has a gauge, which indicates the amount of oxygen remaining. Your baby's doctor will prescribe the flow rate in liters per minute.

The hospital will provide you with a portable tank to get home. Your first oxygen delivery is typically the day of discharge. A respiratory technologist (RT) who works for the oxygen supply company will explain the mechanics of changing the regulator, but it's a good idea to spend some time with an RT in the hospital and have them show you how to change a tank before your baby is discharged.

To go home on oxygen, you must:

- Be able to replace the sticky patches on the side of the head that hold the oxygen tubing in place.
- Know the flow rate and how to set it.

- Be able to read the gauge and know when to switch to a new tank.
- Be comfortable switching the regulator to a full tank.
- Understand the special precautions of living with oxygen, which is very flammable. Always keep the tanks out of direct sunlight, avoid exposing them to temperature extremes, and keep them away from open fire, including cigarettes.

Apnea Monitor and Pulse Oximeter

If your baby is otherwise ready for discharge but is still at risk for apnea (pauses in breathing) or episodic drops in the oxygen level (oxygen desaturation), a monitor will be needed. There are two options for monitors. The first is an apnea monitor, which is attached to a belt around the chest that detects movement. If there are no breathing movements, the alarm will sound. (It's typically set to sound after 20 seconds.) The other option is a pulse oximeter, a version of the one your baby has been attached to for her entire hospitalization. (See chapter 6.) The pulse oximeter records oxygen saturation and heart rate. It is set to alarm if the oxygen saturation falls below a certain level.

Car Seats

There seem to be an endless number of car seats. Having a good fit is essential, not only to keep your baby as safe as possible but to prevent her from slumping over and kinking off her airway. A baby is positioned correctly in her car seat when she is centered and the straps can be tightened so that nothing larger than one of your fingers can slip between the straps and the baby. Almost 25 percent of premature infants do not fit well into the car seat their parent brings to the NICU.

Choose a car seat with these characteristics to get the best fit for your baby:

- **Appropriate weight limits.** Most car seats are only rated for a baby five pounds or larger. If your baby weighs less than five pounds, you will need a car seat with a lower weight limit of four pounds.
- **A five-point harness,** which has straps that go over the shoulders, over the thighs, and between the legs, providing a snugger fit than a three-point system (straps over the shoulders and between the legs).
- **No safety shield,** which is a plastic tray that is part of some harness systems. They are less secure and can injure your baby in an accident.
- **A harness that can give the tightest fit.** A premature baby has less muscle tone and can easily slump to one side. The best option is a shoulder harness that can be lowered to eight inches or less and a seat with a shorter distance from the back of the car seat to the crotch strap.

Even with all these considerations, almost every premature baby needs some kind of padding to get the safest fit. To keep a baby centered and straight, the recommendation from the National Center for Safe Transportation of Children with Special Medical Needs is to pad the sides, around the top of the head, and between the legs with a total of three to four receiving blankets tightly rolled to 5 to 6.5 cm (2 to 2½ inches) in diameter. Pad the sides first to keep your baby centered, and then bend the third receiving blanket around the outside of the side rolls and the head to keep the neck straight. At this point, check the fit. If there's a gap of more than one finger between your baby and the crotch strap, the fourth roll should be placed between the legs with the bend at the crotch (Figure 12). Do not use any device that's not made by the manufacturer specifically for that model to support your baby's head. If a baby cannot stay centered or keeps slumping over despite several attempts with blanket rolls, it's time to consider a different model and start the fit process over again. Brand-specific information about car seat weight limits and harness height can be found at www.preemieprimer.com.

FIGURE 12: Optimal Car Seat Positioning

A. rolls along each side

B. roll over top

C. roll bent between legs

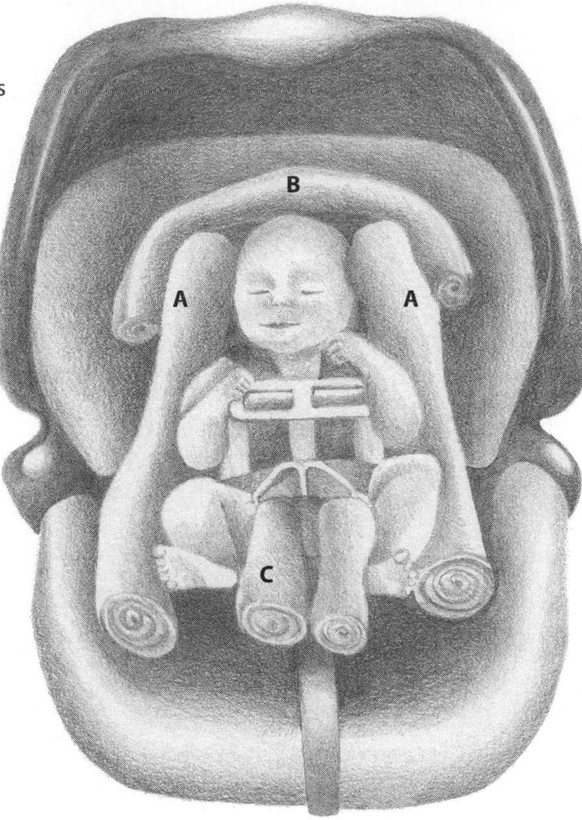

Car Seat Challenge Test

Almost every newborn baby has periodic drops in oxygen while in a car seat, and by two hours in a car seat, more than 15 percent of term babies have significant reductions in their oxygen level. This is an even bigger concern for premature babies, because low muscle tone makes them more prone to postures that can kink off the airway. Premature lungs may also be less able to tolerate a drop in oxygen level. For these reasons, the American Academy of Pediatrics recommends testing the oxygen level and heart rate for 90 minutes in the car seat to be sure they are adequate before a premature baby goes home.

If your baby does not pass the car seat challenge, it's almost always due to position, so repositioning your baby as well as placing the car seat in its most reclined angle (generally 45 degrees) often helps. If these changes don't work, the options are to try a different car seat or to re-evaluate your baby's readiness for discharge.

Some people advocate car beds, vehicle restraint devices that allow a baby to lie flat, if a premature baby does not pass a car seat challenge. However, oxygen levels also drop in car beds, and 19 percent of premature babies will not pass a car bed challenge. The reason is unknown, but unless specifically recommended there's probably no advantage to a car bed over a car seat.

The Mechanics of Going Home

An infant car seat is rear facing, so it's impossible for the driver to see a baby's face. This is stressful enough for any new parent, but maintaining correct positioning in a car seat is even more important for a premature baby. In addition, babies who require supplemental oxygen should be observed to make sure their nasal prongs stay in place. Someone should sit in the back seat to watch your baby's position and her oxygen prongs. Mirror systems, devices that allow the driver to see a rear-facing baby in

Looking back on pictures from those first few months at home, I'm aghast at how my boys actually fit (or rather didn't fit) into the car seats. They were slumped to one side, necks kinked off, with unapproved inserts. I had no idea about blanket rolls, and it never occurred to me to lower the harness. And our car seat was rated to five pounds, yet both boys didn't reach that mark until several weeks after discharge. To top it all off, we had two backseat mirrors rigged up for almost a year.

We thought we were doing our best, but we were swayed by store displays and bought without really thinking. Now I think everything through, because something designed for a term baby may not work for a premature baby. And even more important, just because a product appears on the store shelves doesn't mean it's safe for your baby, regardless of her gestational age.

the rearview mirror, are not recommended. They are distracting for the driver, potentially increasing the risk of an accident, and can dislodge in an accident, injuring your baby.

For some parents, air travel is the fastest way home from the NICU. Airplanes are pressurized to 8,000 feet, a noticeable reduction in oxygen compared to sea level. Many premature babies will need supplemental oxygen to fly, and babies on oxygen may need a higher flow rate. Discuss your travel plans with the medical team so they can make the right recommendations. However, flying with oxygen is not as simple as taking a tank on the plane. Oxygen is a potential explosive hazard, so most airlines have restrictions and/or extra charges. Airlines can change policies and prices, so get airline-specific information a few weeks before you plan to travel. A good resource is the Airline Oxygen Council (link on www.preemieprimer.com). There are also private organizations, charities, and individuals who offer private aircraft and pilot services, and they may be more flexible with oxygen. Many NICUs have regular contacts and can help with these arrangements.

Prescriptions

Many premature babies need medications at home. The following recommendations will help prevent mix-ups and medication errors:

- **Have the prescription sent to the discharge pharmacy the day before discharge** to allow ample time to deal with insurance issues.
- **Speak with a clinical pharmacist** to review the medication(s); ask about potential interactions with other drugs, over-the-counter medications, and food.
- **Insist on written information** about each medication, including dose, how often it should be taken, and potential side effects. Ask what to do if you miss a dose. Instructions are easily misunderstood, so repeat them back to the pharmacist.
- **Ask how to store the medications,** since some need to be kept in the fridge and others should not be exposed to light.

- Mix and administer at least one dose of each medication prior to discharge.
- Ask for the largest supply of medication, although typically only a 30-day supply is allowed with a discharge medication.

Follow-up Appointments

The first appointment will generally be within seven days of discharge. Your baby may also need an eye appointment in her first week or two at home as well as appointments with other specialists. Make sure you have *all* these appointments set up at least a day or two before discharge. Your baby's nurse or social worker will help you. If you have an HMO and your baby needs to see a specialist, call your baby's primary care provider to get the referral and then call your insurance to get the authorization number. The last thing you want is to show up for your baby's first appointment with a specialist and find out there are insurance issues.

CPR Certification

CPR, or cardiopulmonary resuscitation, is a way to keep blood and oxygen flowing in the event the heart stops beating or breathing stops. No one expects to need CPR, but having a medically fragile baby increases the risk. Being prepared is never a bad idea. Most hospitals have an instructional video; however, a CPR course is even better. Your social worker, local Red Cross, or fire department may know of low-cost or free courses.

Home Health

The social worker will know what home services your insurance provides as well as which services are available through federal, state, and county programs. It's wise to use every resource, especially physical and/or occupational therapy, as often these services are limited by health insurance plans.

That first night, Tony and I just stared at Oliver in the bassinet. We were so happy; it was hard to believe he was actually home. The problem? Oliver didn't seem so thrilled. He fussed and fussed. In the NICU he had been unflappable, but now he was inconsolable. We ran through a checklist: he was fed, dry, and comfortable, and had a good oxygen level, but something was still wrong. At 2 AM, Tony gave up and went to bed. I kept trying: I held him, rocked him, walked with him, but he still fussed and cried. Around 3 AM, I too gave up and turned on the TV. It was like a drug—within minutes he was fast asleep. So used to the noise of the NICU, he found the silence at home unnerving. I'd like to say we have weaned him off the TV, but unfortunately it's still his favorite treat. If I had it to do all over, I would have picked classical music!

Transferring to a Hospital Closer to Home

Many babies in an NICU are far from home. As your baby's medical condition improves, she may be medically stable enough to be transferred to a level II nursery closer to your home. This is called **back transport.** Babies who are transferred to a level II nursery grow and do as well developmentally as babies who stay in the NICU. The neonatologists know the surrounding level II nurseries and will not recommend a transfer if they have concerns. Things to consider about back transport include the following:

- **Is the nursery NIDCAP certified?** If not, reconsider. Babies have the best prognosis when they receive this kind of specialized care. (See chapter 8.)
- **Is there a qualified opthalmologist for eye exams** and laser surgery if needed?
- **Check your health insurance** to find out if the ambulance ride is a covered benefit and if there is a co-payment for admission to the new hospital. If your baby has Medicaid, this should not be an issue.

20

Primary Care

The first step in organizing your baby's medical care at home is to identify a primary care provider (PCP). There are several choices: neonatologist, pediatrician, family doctor, and nurse practitioner (NP). A PCP provides all of your baby's basic medical care as well as referrals to specialists. The ideal PCP has a lot of experience with premature babies, is kind, can help with insurance problems, and listens to your concerns.

Premature babies have a lot of office visits, so you also want to consider practicalities, such as how easy it is to get hold of someone when you have questions, appointment availability, the distance of the office from your home, and parking. You also want to know who provides coverage when your baby's PCP is unavailable. If you have an HMO, the right choice is even more important because you cannot access specialists without pre-authorization from the PCP. (See chapter 16.)

Some neonatologists continue to see premature babies after discharge, often in a special NICU follow-up clinic staffed with other health care professionals such as respiratory therapists, physical therapists, social workers, and nutritionists. Many premature babies have complex medical needs, so a medical team all in one place can be helpful. The downside of seeing a neonatologist is that there are times when they are committed to working in the NICU, so there may be less flexibility with appointment times. Because neonatologists are specialists, many HMOs refuse to recognize them as primary care providers, so insurance issues can arise. There may also be travel logistics, as most neonatologists are in larger cities.

There are many excellent pediatricians, family physicians, and nurse practitioners who will also provide your baby with excellent care. An advantage to this is that you begin to feel as though you are entering "normal parenthood." Pediatricians, family doctors, and nurse practitioners are all recognized as PCPs, making this option far easier from an insurance standpoint.

Start thinking about a PCP once your baby has moved to an open crib. Ask the doctors and nurse practitioners in the hospital whom they recommend. They often know many local providers who care for premature and medically fragile children and who might be suited to your baby's unique needs. Connect with other parents—a good recommendation from someone you trust, who has already been there, is invaluable.

If you choose a PCP you've never met, call and ask for a "getting to know the doctor" appointment. This is a chance to address your concerns without the physical distraction of caring for your baby. It's also an opportunity to check out the physical facilities, such as the waiting room and parking, and a good time to gauge your interactions with the office staff, especially the insurance coordinator.

Practical Points about Follow-up Care

There will be detailed instructions and complex information at every appointment. You will also have a lot of questions. If your baby was less than 32 weeks at birth, you can plan on 20 or so visits to your PCP alone in the first year, never mind eye appointments, physical therapy, or specialist visits. This is a lot to coordinate and process. To keep on top of things, start a medical care binder for your baby—a date book or portable desk calendar works well, especially if there are pockets for receipts, loose bits of paper, and business cards (take a business card from *every* health professional you meet).

Plan for each medical appointment. Think about the reason for the appointment (regular checkup, a new problem, or the first appointment with a specialist) and your concerns, no matter how small or silly they might seem. Small things are sometimes early warning signs of larger problems. Because it's easy to get flustered when talking with medical professionals (even for mothers who are also doctors), write down your questions in advance. Consider rehearsing them at home, because questions can sound completely different out loud than they do in your head.

To help remember all the important things for each visit with the PCP, try using this pneumonic—*preemie age*:

- Progress, both physical and behavioral milestones
- Respiratory function
- Eyes
- Ears or hearing
- Medications
- Infection prevention
- Eating and nutrition
- Appointments
- Growth
- Extra

Victor was admitted to the hospital when he was 20 months old with a cold. While we were in the hospital, one of the nurses asked, "Does he always snore like that?" His snoring was already legendary in our house. In the back of my mind, I wondered if perhaps he had sleep apnea (pauses in breathing during sleep), and I *meant* to discuss this at almost every doctor's appointment, but somehow I was always side-tracked by oxygen levels, eating problems, or some other issue. Sure enough, that was exactly what was happening. His tonsils and adenoids were massive and blocking his airway when he was sleeping.

Surgeons removed Victor's tonsils and adenoids, and my husband and I were amazed. Even with the swelling from the surgery, he was so quiet and slept so well we couldn't believe it. Sitting by his hospital bed that night I designed my "preemie" pneumonic, so I would (hopefully) never forget to ask my questions again.

Progress

Your baby's PCP should ask you about your baby's development at each visit (see chapter 26 for specific developmental milestones) and discuss any of your concerns about development. Specific screening tests are performed at the nine-month, 18-month, and 30-month visit (although not all insurances pay for a 30-month visit, so the third screen might happen at 24 months). A screen for autism is performed at 18 and 24 months. Developmental screening is initially based on your baby's adjusted age, but when she reaches the age of two, her unadjusted age is used.

Respiratory Function

Many premature babies will have their oxygen level checked at each visit. How long this continues will depend on your baby's lungs, if she's been sick, and if she's on oxygen. Your PCP will ask about secondhand smoke, which increases the risk of asthma and doubles the risk of a hospital admission due to infection.

Eyes

In certain cases, follow-up with an ophthalmologist is needed:

- **Your baby had ROP that required treatment.** Close follow-up is needed to identify any residual problems that may require correction. The ophthalmologist will also prescribe glasses if needed.
- **Your baby has immature blood vessels or stage 1 or 2 ROP.** Surveillance is needed until the blood vessels in the eyes mature or the ROP resolves. This can take several weeks or even months after discharge home. In addition, a screening exam is recommended at six months, one year, and two years of age.

Premature babies also have an increased incidence of myopia (nearsightedness), strabismus (crossed eyes), and amblyopia (lazy eye). This is unrelated to ROP. To screen for these problems, all premature babies should have an appointment with an ophthalmologist between six and nine months (adjusted age). A vision check with the PCP at the age of three and again at four years of age is also recommended.

Ears

If your baby did not pass the newborn screening, she should be evaluated within three months by an audiologist (hearing expert) for more precise testing. If hearing loss is confirmed, services should begin as early as possible, preferably before your baby is six months old, because early intervention improves language skills and communication.

Speak up if you are concerned about your baby's hearing. One study showed that parents identify hearing impairment earlier than their child's pediatrician does. Reasons your baby should have her hearing tested include:

- **Repeated ear infections with persistent fluid in the ears.**
- **Your baby does not seem to respond to sound.**
- **Delay in language skills.**

A language delay may be the result of a hearing impairment, but it can also be a symptom of a sensory processing disorder, a weakness of facial muscles, a more overall delay, or another medical condition. The minimal language milestones are listed in Table 1. While your doctor may feel your baby needs an evaluation earlier, if your baby is not meeting these milestones make sure to ask for a referral to the appropriate specialist. If the concern is hearing, your baby should see an audiologist and a pediatric ear, nose, and throat (ENT) specialist. If the concern involves weakness, sensory issues, or delays in other areas of development, such as motor milestones, referral to a pediatric neurologist may be appropriate. Regardless of the cause, if your baby is two years old or older and has delays in speech, referreral to a speech therapist is recommended.

TABLE 1: Language Milestones

Adjusted age	Language
By 6 months	Turns head to sounds; watches your face when you speak; laughs, giggles, cries, or fusses; makes noise when talked to
By 12 months	Babbles ("ba-ba-ba" or "ma-ma-ma"), understands "no-no," tries to imitate sounds, tries to communicate by actions or gestures
By 18 months	Follows simple directions accompanied by gestures; points to objects, pictures, and family members; answers simple questions nonverbally, tries to imitate simple words
By 24 months	Points to simply body parts (such as "nose"), says 40 words (pronunciation may be unclear), asks for common foods by name, says "mine," makes animal sounds such as "moo"
By 36 months	Knows name, age, sex, colors; can speak in 2- to 3-word sentences, speech is 75 percent intelligible, asks "W" questions (when, what, where, why)
By 4 years	Correctly names colors, speaks in sentences of 5 or 6 words, tells stories, knows basic grammar rules, strangers can understand most of what is said
By 5 years	Understands time sequences (what came first, second, and third), understands rhyming, speaks in sentences of 8 or more words, engages in conversation, can remember and retell part of a story, understands more than 2,000 words

Neither of my boys said a word before the age of two. Every day I hoped this would be the day I'd hear "Mama." There was cooing and babbling, but no words. Eventually Victor started speaking, but Oliver was behind. I was convinced he was hearing impaired or had some other delay. Tony just shook his head. "He's ignoring us," he said.

"How do you know?" I challenged. "Did they teach auditory processing in architecture school?"

"It's a guy thing," he said with a shrug.

So off we went for the testing. We sat together in a room while beeps and whistles emerged from different corners. Oliver responded correctly to every single one.

We were both right. Oliver's hearing was fine, but he had a speech delay. We did speech therapy, the Hannon program, and special education with the school district for a year. And we had many detailed but one-sided conversations where he would just listen and laugh and laugh, but not say much. Then, when he was three and a half, it was as if the gears clicked and suddenly he couldn't stop talking!

My Oliver is a crafty one. To this day he is skilled at selective listening. He never hears me when I ask him to pick up his clothes, but I can whisper at the other end of the house about buying a toy and suddenly I am tripping all over him. Sometimes it has as much to do with personality as prematurity.

Medications

Review medications at every visit. Take the actual bottles to avoid errors transcribing names and doses. It's a hassle, but many medications sound very similar, and moving the decimal point one place can have major ramifications.

Your baby will grow rapidly, especially in the first few months. Ask if medication doses need to be readjusted based on a change in weight. Also be honest if you're having problems remembering to give a medication. *It's hard to do it all, all of the time.* Sometimes regimens can be simplified, and if taste is an issue, another formulation may be possible.

Infection Prevention

Vaccines are a very important part of your baby's preventive care. Make sure to keep track of all her vaccines so you know she is up-to-date. When your baby is premature, she is more vulnerable to infections, and if she gets sick, the consequences may be more severe. Many parents have detailed questions about vaccines, so this subject is covered in depth in chapter 21.

Eating

Premature babies require extra calories to support their catch-up growth. Additional medical challenges, like lung and heart problems, further increase their caloric requirements. If you are breast-feeding, keep track of how often your baby nurses and report any difficulties or concerns. If your baby is bottle-fed, do a 24-hour log before your appointments so you know the volume she is eating. Track any solids as well. If your baby is not growing as expected, her PCP needs to know if insufficient calorie intake is playing a role.

If your baby is being fed a formula designed for a premature baby, the protein, vitamin, and mineral balance will be just right. Breast-fed babies, however, require a vitamin D supplement, and if they're too old for a human milk fortifier with iron, they may also require an iron supplement. Ask about supplements at every visit.

Discuss any feeding problems, such as refusing to eat or spitting up. If your baby is tube fed, ask about plans to transition to oral feeds.

Do not introduce solids (including cereals) until you get the go-ahead from your baby's PCP. Solid foods have fewer calories and nutrients than breast milk or formula and may not support your baby's nutritional needs. Also, your baby is not physically ready to attempt solids until she has good head control, which may take longer for a premature baby than for a baby born at term.

My height has defined my life. I was always the tallest. It was my super-power. It gave me confidence. I always believed my height helped me to compete in the male-dominated world of surgery. In my day, male surgeons loved to make female medical students and residents stand on step stools at the operating table. At 5 feet 10½ inches, I stood as tall as, if not taller than, the surgeons. I am above the 95th percentile for height.

I didn't think much about Oliver and Victor's size at first. There was too much else going on, and we were feeding them as much as they could eat. I became acutely aware of their petite statures when they started kinder-garten and Oliver was still wearing size 2 pants. Victor, propelled by his love of all things chocolate, had managed to squeak up to the 25th percentile, but Oliver, drained by bad lungs, a bad heart, and God knows what else, is barely at the 5th percentile for weight and the 10th percentile for height. Plotting him out on the growth curve, Oliver will be 5 feet 6 inches, a lot shorter than his genetically predicted height of 6 feet 1 inches.

I used to obsess over those 7 inches. All the unfairness of prematurity, and I'm worried about height? And then I started to think about how height has affected my brother. He is 6 feet 2 inches and is as shy as I am gregarious. Where I flaunted my height, he wished he could be shorter. His only desire was to fit in; mine was to stand out. And that is, of course, when it all made sense. My height has not defined my life, but rather my life has defined my height. I need to make sure that's the message I pass on to my boys.

Appointments

Before you leave the office, make sure you set up the next appointment. Ask if letters from specialists have been received and inquire about any specialist appointments that may be needed, such as physical therapy or speech therapy.

Growth

How well your baby is growing and gaining weight is a good indicator of her health and nutrition. Growth, weight, and head circumference will be plotted on a growth curve using adjusted age until your baby is two years old. After age two, the unadjusted age will be used. Where your baby's height and weight are at a given point in time (for example, the 10th percentile or 50th percentile) is not as important as *how* she is gaining in length and weight. Use the growth curve in the appendix or download one from www.preemieprimer.com to track your baby's progress for your own records. (Growth curves are gender specific, so make sure you use the right one.)

Extras

A reminder to discuss any additional problems and ask questions not answered during the appointment. This is another reason why it's a good idea to plan and rehearse. Think about what has happened since the last appointment, review any notes you have made about your concerns, and organize your questions.

21

Infection Control

Infection is the number one reason a premature baby will be re-admitted to the hospital. Weaker immune systems, nutritional problems, and damaged lungs increase the risk a premature baby will catch an infection if exposed. In addition, premature babies are more likely to suffer significant consequences of an infection. What might be a minor illness for an adult or even a term baby can be devastating, especially in the first few years. The most concerning infections involve the lungs. These infections can cause more lung injury and delay healing from the effects of prematurity.

Preventing infection is an essential part of your baby's care. It's hard to know how long your baby will be more prone to infections. Degree of prematurity, weight, nutritional intake, residual lung issues, and other illnesses all play a role. However, with time, lungs heal and immune systems strengthen, so as your baby gets older she should become more resilient.

Hand Hygiene

Maintain the same hand hygiene rituals at home that you used in the hospital. Keep several bottles of alcohol-based hand sanitizer around the house, including one at the front door to catch people on their way in. Also keep one in the diaper bag. Insist that everyone, yourself included, use sanitizer or wash their hands well, before touching your baby.

One big source of germs in a doctor's office is the pen given to you at check-in to complete forms—it has probably touched hundreds of people, many of whom were sick, and has never been cleaned. Keep several pens in your diaper bag, and always use your own.

Limit Contact

It's hard to stay away from people when your baby comes home from the hospital. You will have many friends who want to come over, and you naturally want to show off your baby. However, people mean germs. Obviously you'll ask someone who is ill to stay away, but you never really know, because people are contagious for two or three days before they feel and look sick. While anyone can transmit an infection, children in day care, their parents, and health care workers pose the greatest risk. This is simply based on the odds of being exposed.

Avoid Secondhand Smoke

The toxins in secondhand smoke damage the airways. Children who are exposed to secondhand smoke are more likely to catch infections and are twice as likely to be admitted to the hospital with a respiratory tract infection.

Vaccinations

A vaccination is a medication designed to stimulate the immune system to make antibodies, which protect against infection. There are several kinds of vaccines:

- **A killed vaccine.** This is an injection of part of a dead virus or bacteria, which is no longer infectious.
- **A live vaccine,** which is made from a virus that has been weakened (also called attenuated). Bacteria cannot be used for a live vaccine. These vaccines are very safe. Rarely, the weakened virus mutates

(changes) and becomes infectious. If this happens, the infection will be much less severe than if the virus had been acquired naturally. Live vaccines are not used in the first year of life or during pregnancy. Only three live vaccines are routinely given in childhood: MMR (measles, mumps, and rubella), chicken pox, and the flu nasal spray.

- **A toxoid vaccine.** Some bacteria cause illness through poisons called toxins. A toxoid vaccine immunizes your baby by using a weakened toxin called a toxoid. Diphtheria and tetanus vaccines are toxoids.

- **An antibody vaccine.** This is a different type of immunization altogether. Technically, it's immunoprophylaxis, an injection of antibodies, the actual disease-fighting weapon. However, for simplicity, it's fine to refer to it as a vaccine. Because these antibodies disappear quickly, the injection needs to be given every month to keep the levels high enough.

Some people have wondered about a potential link between autism and vaccines, focusing specifically on a vaccine component called thimerosal. It *is* important to have a critical eye for every medical decision, and vaccines are no different. The incidence of autism is higher among premature babies, and no parent wants to do anything that could increase the risk.

Thimerosal is a preservative used in the manufacturing process of some vaccines and contains ethyl mercury. This is not the same as methyl mercury, which is found in dental fillings and fish. Thimerosal may cause minor reactions at the injection site, like swelling or redness, but there is no medical evidence that the small amount of thimerosal in vaccines has ever posed any risk. Furthermore, thimerosal was removed from all pediatric vaccines in 2001. (It's present in a few adult vaccines such as diphtheria, tetanus, and some influenza vaccines.) Despite removing thimerosal, there has been no drop in autism rates in the past eight years. There are also many studies published in respected medical journals showing *there is no link between thimerosal or vaccines and autism.*

Why was thimerosal removed if it's safe? Back when the initial concerns were raised, these studies had not been performed. Now we know for sure that it's not a concern, and removing chemicals from medications is never a bad thing if it doesn't compromise the effectiveness. The biggest risks with vaccines are minor effects like swelling and redness at the injection site. The stimulation of the immune system may also cause your child to run a low-grade fever for a day or so.

Vaccine refusal by parents is increasing, and in turn, so are potentially dangerous vaccine-preventable diseases. Outbreaks of measles, rubella, and pertussis (whooping cough) are the highest they have been in years. These diseases are not benign for any child, but are especially concerning for a premature baby. When other parents refuse to vaccinate their children, they increase the chances that your baby will get sick from one of these infections. Your baby is not fully protected by her vaccines until she is 18 months old. In addition, while vaccines dramatically reduce your baby's risk of many serious infections, they are not 100 percent effective—a *small* percentage will still get sick. However, the antibodies generated by vaccination reduce the severity of the illness.

Influenza

The flu, or seasonal influenza, is a virus that infects millions every year. A lot of people mistakenly refer to a runny nose or a cold as the flu, but

Oliver received every childhood vaccine and was still hospitalized twice with vaccine-preventable diseases, including once in the intensive care unit. Some people ask me why I still get him immunized, because vaccines "obviously don't work for him."

I look at it from an entirely different perspective. No medical treatment is 100 percent effective. Statistically, however, a child who is vaccinated is less likely to get sick. If they do get sick, they're less likely to be seriously ill.

Oliver has the bad heart, bad lungs, and bad immune system trifecta. Without his vaccinations, he might have died. I'll take all the help I can get.

the flu is much more serious. Colds are generally mild, and while they're annoying, they don't pose a significant health hazard. Influenza, on the other hand, causes a higher fever, extreme tiredness, and muscle aches. It can also cause pneumonia (infection of the lungs) and kills more than 35,000 people in the United States every year. Children under the age of five, pregnant women, and people with chronic health problems, especially heart and lung conditions, are more likely to have serious complications. More than 20,000 children are hospitalized every year because of influenza. A premature baby is at significant risk for influenza-related complications.

Unlike other vaccine-preventable diseases, seasonal influenza changes slightly every year, so the antibodies to last year's influenza will not be effective against this year's strains. That's why a new vaccine is needed every year. The Centers for Disease Control and Prevention (CDC) recommends annual vaccination for seasonal influenza once your baby is six months old (unadjusted age). The first time your baby is vaccinated, she will need two doses 28 days apart.

A new strain of influenza called H1N1 (or swine flu) is also circulating. Like seasonal influenza, H1N1 can produce serious infections. Premature babies are among the most vulnerable. Starting in the fall of 2010 the plan is to combine H1N1 with the seasonal influenza vaccine.

The seasonal influenza and H1N1 vaccinations are available by injection or in a nasal spray. The injection is a killed virus and the nasal spray is a live, weakened virus. Your baby cannot receive the nasal spray until she is two years old. People with asthma also should not receive the nasal spray, as even a weakened virus can potentially irritate vulnerable airways. After vaccination with the nasal spray, small amounts of the weakened virus can spread to 1 to 2 percent of household contacts. As the virus is very weak, it's unlikely to produce actual influenza; however, if your premature baby is still too young to be vaccinated, play it safe and have people in your household vaccinated with an injection.

As a doctor, I'm very critical of every therapy. Medications, including vaccines, have to be backed up by good science *and* the benefits must clearly outweigh the risks. I'm not about to give my boys anything that is dangerous. I didn't get them through the NICU to risk autism or any other health problem from a vaccine.

It's hard when your child is ill. It's even harder when no one has identified a reason. My boys don't have autism, but they have other serious and unexplained medical conditions such as congenital heart disease, bronchopulmonary dysplasia, hypothyroidism, and cerebral palsy. I can't presume to understand what a parent with an autistic child faces, but I understand something about having a child with a chronic and largely untreatable medical condition. It's a difficult road, made more challenging by not understanding the "why." If someone offers you something concrete to blame, it's hard to ignore.

The autism-vaccine theory has been disproved. I have scoured the scientific articles, and I have no safety concerns. As a doctor I have also seen patients get very sick from vaccine-preventable diseases and have seen some die. Most had weakened immune systems, but some were young and healthy. One was a healthy 25-year-old girl, the same age as I was at the time.

My generation and many before me received the smallpox vaccine. It left a decent-size scar. It was a mandatory part of the global fight against smallpox. I grew up in Winnipeg and realistically there was probably a greater chance of being struck by a meteor than getting smallpox. But we were all vaccinated. Because I have that scar, my children don't have to worry about smallpox. That is the power of a vaccine—the ability to protect one person and everyone, especially the most vulnerable. I feel proud when I get vaccinated, because I know I'm not helping only myself.

Respiratory Syncyctial Virus (RSV)

RSV is a common respiratory tract infection. For most people it causes a moderate to severe cold that lasts for one to two weeks. RSV can also cause mucus buildup and inflammation in the airways (bronchiolitis) as well as pneumonia. (See chapter 22.) Babies, who have smaller airways and a weaker immune system, are at greater risk for complications. RSV is very serious for premature babies.

The RSV vaccine is called *palivizumab* or *Synagis*. It reduces your baby's chance of needing to be hospitalized due to an RSV infection. RSV shots start in the late fall (as RSV is almost never seen before December) and continue to the spring, when the infection disappears. The RSV season is typically about five months, but the time it starts may vary slightly depending on where you live. Because the RSV shot is not a true vaccine but an injection of protective antibodies (immunoprophylaxis), it only lasts for one month and must be given monthly during RSV season to maintain protection. Indications for *Synagis* are based on the risk for hospitalization associated with RSV infection:

- **Premature children less than two years of age with chronic lung disease who receive medical therapy for bronchopulmonary dysplasia (such as oxygen, inhalers, or steroid medication) or congenital heart disease** will receive five doses their first year and up to five doses their second season.
- **Premature infants who were less than 28[6] weeks and are less than 12 months old at the start of RSV season** may receive up to five doses in their first RSV season.
- **Premature infants who were born between 29 and 31[6] weeks and are less than six months old at the start of RSV season** may receive up to five doses in their first RSV season.
- **Premature infants born between 32 and 34[6] weeks who are less than three months old at the start of RSV season and at high risk for RSV** (and either attend day care or have a brother or sister younger than five years of age) will receive up to three doses in their first RSV season.

Getting *Synagis* approved can be an insurance hassle, because it costs about $900 a shot. If your baby meets the criteria listed above, the first step is to make sure RSV prevention is a covered benefit, and the second step is to obtain pre-authorization. The paperwork will be submitted by your baby's doctor, but be proactive and call your insurance company to check on the pre-authorization status.

Because the RSV immunization is given once a month, you will either need to take your baby to the doctor's office during RSV season for every injection or a nurse will come to your house—this decision is dictated by your insurance company. If the injection is given at home, call your pharmacy several days beforehand so they can make sure it's in stock and to double check that there have been no insurance issues.

If you don't have insurance, your baby may be eligible to receive *Synagis* at no cost from the manufacturer's patient assistance program (MedImmune). Specific information about working out the insurance hassles of *Synagis* and the patient assistance program is available at www.preemieprimer.com.

Whooping Cough

Whooping cough is a respiratory infection caused by the bacteria **pertussis.** It starts the way a common cold does, with runny nose or congestion, sneezing, a mild cough, and fever. After one to two weeks, the symptoms change and severe coughing begins. Children with the disease may cough violently and rapidly, over and over, until the air is gone from their lungs and they're forced to inhale with a loud "whooping" sound.

Pertussis is a serious infection for children: 10 percent get pneumonia, 2 percent will have seizures, and more than 50 percent of babies under the age of one will need to be hospitalized. Pertussis can also cause inflammation around the brain. The risk of dying is 1 in 1,000. Pertussis is given as part of the DTaP vaccine, which is a three-in-one vaccine: diphtheria, tetanus (lockjaw), and pertussis. Five doses of DTaP are given before kindergarten: at two, four, six, and 15 to 18 months and again at four to six years.

An unvaccinated baby is 23 times more likely to catch pertussis than a baby who has been vaccinated. Pertussis is now the most common vaccine-preventable disease, as more parents decline vaccinations for their children. Currently there are about 10,000 cases of pertussis every year in the United States.

Other Vaccine-preventable Diseases

Immunization is also recommended against:

- **Haemophilus influenzae type b (HiB),** a bacterial infection that can cause meningitis (infection of the membranes that cover the brain and spinal cord) and pneumonia. Vaccination requires four doses at two, four, six, and 12 to 15 months.
- **Chicken pox,** which is a fever and itchy rash caused by the varicella zoster virus (VZV). It can also cause infection of the brain or the lungs (pneumonia). It requires two vaccinations, one given at 12 to 15 months and again at four to six years. If a pregnant mother catches chicken pox, her baby is at risk for serious health problems.
- **Measles,** or infection with the rubeola virus. It can cause fever, cough, runny nose, and a rash. It can also lead to pneumonia and inflammation of the brain (encephalitis). One to three children out of every 1,000 children who get measles will die. Measles vaccine is given as part of the two-dose MMR (measles, mumps, rubella) vaccine series at 12 to 15 months and at four to six years.
- **Mumps,** a viral illness that causes swelling of the salivary glands in the cheek. Complications include inflammation of the brain (encephalitis) and of the membranes that line the brain (meningitis), deafness, and damage to the testicles. The mumps vaccine is given as part of the MMR vaccine.
- **Rubella,** also called the German measles, which is a virus that causes a rash, slight fever, and enlarged lymph nodes. The disease is often mild; however, if a pregnant mother is exposed, her baby runs a 20 percent chance of developing serious birth defects. Rubella vaccine is part of the MMR vaccine.
- **Pneumococcus,** a bacteria that causes pneumonia, ear infections, sinusitis, and meningitis. The vaccine is given at two, four, six, and 12 to 15 months.

- **Hepatitis A and B,** viruses that infect the liver. The hepatitis A vaccine is given at one year and again at age two. Hepatitis B vaccine is given at birth, with a second dose at one to two months and a third between six and 18 months.
- **Polio,** a virus that invades the nervous system. One percent of those infected with polio will be permanently paralyzed. The vaccine is given at two, four, and six months and a booster at four to six years.

22

~~~~~~~~~~~~~~~~~

Lungs at Home

A term baby has 30 to 50 million alveoli (air sacs). However, production of alveoli skyrockets after birth, and by age eight, the lungs have about 300 million alveoli. A premature baby has much fewer alveoli at birth compared with a term baby, but the capacity to produce new alveoli at such a rapid rate allows the lungs to heal with time. Most children improve dramatically as they and their lungs grow. During this time, you'll need to promote adequate nutrition to optimize lung repair (see chapter 23), and it will be essential to avoid the two factors most likely to injure the recovering and vulnerable lungs: cigarette smoke and infections.

Bronchopulmonary Dysplasia (BPD)

BPD is a disease characterized by structural changes in the lung that result from a premature delivery, specifically fewer alveoli with thicker walls, which affects oxygen transfer from the lungs to the blood. Inflammation is also a component. Interruption of normal lung development before birth is the biggest risk factor for BPD. The earlier the interruption, the greater the risk—20 percent of babies born before 30 weeks will develop BPD. Other factors that affect a baby's risk of BPD include:

- **Infection,** both before and after delivery.
- **Need for oxygen**—how much and for how long.

- **Length of time on a ventilator.**
- **Genetic factors.**

Many babies with BPD will need supplemental oxygen when they come home. While daunting at first, managing with home oxygen quickly becomes part of your normal routine. (See chapter 19.) Don't be alarmed if the amount of oxygen is gradually increased, because babies with BPD may need more oxygen as they grow.

Management of BPD includes:

- **Diuretics (water pill),** medication that keeps a baby slightly dehydrated. BPD-affected lungs are often leaky, allowing excess fluid to accumulate around the air sacs, which makes it harder to breathe. A diuretic helps get rid of this fluid. How long your baby needs to stay on a diuretic will depend on many factors.
- **Maximizing nutrition.** Many babies with BPD will need 50 percent to 100 percent more calories a day. Not only does your baby use more energy to breathe, but the body also uses a lot of calories repairing itself.
- **Avoiding cigarette smoke,** as the toxins will damage your baby's lungs as well as increase her risk for infection.
- **Preventing lung infections,** because each infection causes more damage.

How long your baby will need supplemental oxygen depends on the severity of her lung disease and how she heals. Most children will be off supplemental oxygen by the age of two, and by age eight most children with BPD will be in the lower range of normal, meaning they will manage just fine.

Whether your baby is on oxygen or not, ask for specific guidelines to help you recognize the warning signs of potential breathing problems, such as abnormal respiratory rate, low oxygen saturation, or signs that your baby is working hard to breathe. Ask specifically what to do in these situations. You need to know when you should call the office and when it's an emergency.

A child with BPD is at risk for extreme inflammation and spasm in the airways in response to a cold or a lung infection. Inflammation and spasms narrow the airways, making it harder to breathe. Some babies will wheeze, but there may be significant airway narrowing even if you cannot hear any wheezing. Airway spasm may also occur in response to pollution, breathing cold air, or vigorous exercise when your child is older.

Medications may be needed to treat both inflammation and airway spasm. There's so much individual variation in how these medications are prescribed that it's best to talk with your baby's health care provider about a plan for your particular circumstances. Make sure you know when and how to use each medication. Some of the more common medications include:

- **Steroids,** which rapidly reduce inflammation. They may be taken by mouth or inhaled. They have serious side effects, such as affecting growth and increasing susceptibility to infection, although these risks are negligible with inhaled steroids. The pills and liquid taste awful, and administering them can be a challenge for many parents. Inhaled steroids are particularly helpful during cold and flu season to prevent the excess inflammation that can result from these infections.

- **Bronchodilators.** These are medications that relax the airways and increase the airflow. They may be given by mouth (*theophylline*) or be inhaled (*albuterol, levalbuterol,* and *ipratropium*). *Theophylline* is taken every day as a preventive measure and *albuterol, levalbuterol,* and *ipratropium* (*Atrovent*) are short-acting medications that only last for a few hours. *Albuterol* is frequently mixed with *ipratropium,* and together these medications work even better. *Levalbuterol* (also called *Xopenex*) and *albuterol* are similar medications, so they are not given together. Some babies can become jittery or hyperactive with *albuterol.* This side effect may be less likely with *levalbuterol,* although this medication is much more expensive.

Steroids and bronchodilators can be administered through an **inhaler,** a small device that dispenses a single dose of medication each time the top is pressed. To deliver the medication deep into the airways, inhalation must be coordinated precisely with pressing the top of the inhaler. This is difficult for children under the age of 12, so a younger child will need a spacer, which is a tube with a face mask at one end and the inhaler at the other. Medication is discharged into the spacer and inhaled through the face mask, eliminating the need for special coordination. Allow your baby to inhale two or three times to get the full dose. Wait one minute to allow the medication to penetrate deep into the lungs before doing a second puff.

Tips on caring for your inhaler include:

- **Keep track of the number of doses used** (each puff is one dose) if the inhaler does not have a counter. It's difficult to tell when they're empty.
- **Prime a new inhaler four times** (discharging four puffs) before the first use to get the medication flowing.
- **Prime the inhaler appropriately between uses.** If it hasn't been used in the past three to seven days, prime twice before using, and prime four times if it hasn't been used for more than seven days.
- **Clean the inhaler if it goes more than seven days between each use.** Pull out the medication canister and rinse the plastic mouthpiece in warm water to free up any clogs; otherwise your child may not get any medication with the first few puffs.
- **Make sure all caregivers, including the school, know about these instructions.**

Bronchodilators may also be administered by a **nebulizer,** a machine that turns medication into a fine mist to be inhaled. The medication comes in small, single-dose vials that must be kept out of the light. The medication is placed in a cup-like piece of equipment that is attached to a face mask. The cup is connected by thin tubing to the nebulizer machine, and when the machine is turned on, the medication becomes a vapor that is inhaled through the face mask. The face mask and cup should be rinsed thoroughly with warm water after each use and left to air dry on a clean towel. They should also be soaked at least once a week for 30 minutes in a solution of one part white vinegar and two parts distilled water, and then rinsed well and left to dry. When dry, store the face mask and cup in a clean plastic bag between uses. Disconnect the thin tubing that connects the nebulizer to the medication cup (this tubing should not be washed) and also store it in a clean plastic bag between uses.

Asthma

Asthma is a condition that causes inflammation and spasm of the airways. It may occur as part of an allergic reaction (such as mold or pollen), be triggered by an irritant (like dust or pollution), or occur in response to a virus, cold weather, or exercise. When the airways become narrow, it's harder to breathe. Wheezing may also occur as air squeezes through the narrow passages.

Approximately 18 percent of premature babies will go on to develop asthma, which is about double the typical childhood rate. There are a lot of similarities between asthma and BPD, such as susceptibility to infections, airway inflammation, and spasm. However, unlike in BPD, the alveoli (air sacs) are not involved in asthma.

An asthma attack is a common reason for needing emergency care. It's crucial to have an asthma action plan—discuss with your baby's providers what you should look for and what you should do in case of an asthma attack. Also ask about what warning signs should prompt you to seek emergency care, such as a fast respiratory rate or if you can see the areas between your child's ribs and at the base of her neck pull in when she breathes. (This means she's using more muscles than she should to breathe.) When your child is seven or eight years old, she may be able to use a **peak flow meter.** This handheld device gives information about how well your child can push air out of her lungs (which is an indicator of airway narrowing). It's important to do peak flow measurements when your child is well, because you compare peak flow measurements during an asthma attack to her "healthy" measurements. You should be given a specific action plan depending on the peak flow.

Avoiding triggers is an essential part of asthma, but medications are commonly needed. Steroids and bronchodilators are used for asthma much in the same way that they are used for BPD—to reduce inflammation and open the constricted airways. *Albuterol, levalbuterol,* and *ipratropium* are rescue medications, meaning they're used during an asthma attack; however, your provider may also recommend using them regularly throughout the day. Some children need inhaled steroids every day to keep their inflammation under control, while others only need steroids episodically. A pill called *montelukast sodium (Singulair)* may be helpful for some children. It blocks chemicals in the body called leukotrienes, which can be involved in an asthma attack.

Infections

Infections are a significant concern, especially for babies and children with BPD and/or asthma. More than 50 percent of babies with BPD will be admitted to the hospital in their first year of life with an infection, and 37 percent in their second year. The physical stress of an infection can affect nutrition and impair growth, and the inflammation may further damage vulnerable lungs. The physical strain can also set your baby back developmentally.

The Common Cold

A cold is a viral infection of the nasal passages and throat. It causes mucus buildup (congestion and a runny nose), cough, a sore throat, and a fever up to 38° C (100.4° F). The mucus may be yellow or green—the color is not important. The buildup is part of the body's immune response. Because the inflammation may also affect the tubes that drain the ears, fluid can collect in the middle ear, causing pain and even leading to an ear infection.

Victor caught a cold when he was about 20 months. He was congested with a runny nose, but his sore throat was the biggest problem, because he just *could not* eat. At the time his oral aversion was still very severe. Once his throat started hurting, he refused to swallow.

By the second day we were in the emergency room and he needed to be hydrated with IV fluids. The third day we were back again for more IV fluids, and finally he was admitted to the hospital.

There was some eye rolling from medical professionals and friends. "What do you mean he won't swallow?" or "He'll eat when he's hungry."

Patiently I tried to explain it wasn't that he *wouldn't* eat, he *couldn't*. However, inside I was screaming, "Why don't you try being vomited on for 18 months so you can tell the difference between won't and can't?"

Fortunately, when his pediatrician (who happened to be his neonatologist) stopped by the following morning, he just nodded his head. "Yup, that happens with oral aversion. He'll eat when he can."

After two days of IV fluids, he was able to drink well enough to go home.

The treatment is humidified air to reduce the swelling, comfort measures, and medications like *acetaminophen* (*Tylenol*) or *ibuprofen*. For most babies, a cold is a minor annoyance; however, for a premature baby with BPD or asthma, the cold virus can trigger inflammation and spasm in the airways. Many babies breathe through their mouths when congested, and this may affect oxygen levels if your baby is on supplemental oxygen. The other concern is difficulty feeding, so it's important to pay attention to input and make sure your baby is not losing weight.

Croup

Croup is inflammation of the upper airways. Like a cold, it's caused by a viral infection, most typically parainfluenza virus. Croup starts like a cold, with congestion and a low-grade fever, but swelling around the vocal cords and trachea (windpipe) produces a cough that sounds like a seal barking. The cough is worse at night and may come in waves. Children with smaller airways, such as premature babies, are more likely to get croup. The virus can also irritate the lower airways, leading to inflammation and spasm. A humidifier will suffice at home for many babies, but some will need hospital admission for IV fluids, nutritional support, oxygen, bronchodilators, and steroids.

Bronchiolitis

Bronchiolitis is a viral infection of the smaller airways or bronchioles. The infection leads to inflammation, swelling of the lining of the airways, and

Oliver tires easily, probably because of a combination of his BPD and his ongoing heart issues. And I don't push him, fearful of the lurking specter of cardiac arrest. But when it came time for a walk-a-thon at his elementary school, we signed up. More cautious than most other parents, we walked the quarter-mile laps with the boys. It was a great October day—sunny with a cool breeze—and our laughter was interrupted only by pit stops for ice cream and popsicles.

Engrossed in conversation with a few other parents, we suddenly realized Oliver was nowhere in sight. We panicked. Tony grabbed Victor's hand and I sprinted off as an invisible vise tightened in my chest. Had he collapsed somewhere?

When I rounded the corner of the school I could see him ahead of me. He was running as fast as his tiny little legs could carry him, with his head thrown back, hair whipping in the wind, arms flailing, and smiling as only Oliver can.

I caught up. "Hey Bud, how are you doing?"

"I'm running Momma, I'm running!" And he was. And pretty fast for him.

It was all I could do to stop from dissolving on the spot. Nine and half weeks in the NICU, 12 months on oxygen, two heart surgeries, seven hospitalizations for pneumonia, countless emergency room visits, and hundreds of sleepless nights for me, sitting by his bed giving him breathing treatments, wondering if we should really be in the emergency room. And here he was running.

Oliver ran a mile that day. It was pretty rough the next week. He needed two days off from school to recover. Yet superimposed over all those bad memories are the images of him full of vigor and joy, running down the grass track on that beautiful fall day.

excess mucus in the bronchioles, just the way a cold causes the nasal passages to swell and become blocked. Basically, bronchiolitis is snotty airways. RSV (respiratory syncyctial virus) is the most common cause of bronchiolitis, but influenza and other viruses may also be the cause.

Bronchiolitis causes wheezing and coughing, which seems to be worse at night. If your child has BPD or asthma, the inflammation can trigger airway spasms and the coughing and other symptoms may last much longer, even for weeks. The virus can also travel down to the alveoli (air sacs in the lungs) and cause pneumonia.

Children under the age of two are at greatest risk for complications; however, older children with more severe BPD, asthma, or heart conditions are also at risk. Some will need to be admitted to the hospital because they are eating poorly or need oxygen. Some children may even need a breathing machine such as a CPAP or a ventilator. (See chapter 6.) Besides supporting nutrition and breathing, the treatment of bronchiolitis includes steroids, if there's significant inflammation, and inhaled bronchodilators. Physical therapy of the chest may help loosen secretions.

Pneumonia

Pneumonia is infection of the lungs' alveoli or air sacs. The resulting inflammation can interfere with the ability to transfer oxygen from the lungs to the blood. The airways, too, may become inflamed and constricted. Pneumonia can be caused by a virus or by a bacteria. Bacterial pneumonia is treated with antibiotics and antiviral medication may be used for some kinds of viral pneumonia.

Some premature babies and older children with pneumonia will need to be admitted to the hospital. In addition to antibiotics or antiviral medications, therapies such as IV fluids, oxygen, bronchodilators, chest physical therapy, and steroids can help. Some babies will need a breathing machine.

23

<hr>

Growth and Nutrition

Growth, especially height, is a reflection of overall good health. If the body is not getting enough nutrition, this may also affect the brain's ability to grow. Therefore, your baby's height and weight will be closely monitored and plotted against growth curves from the Centers for Disease Control and Prevention. (See Appendix.) While your baby is under the age of two, head circumference will also be measured. Adjusted age is typically used for the first two years, but after age two only the unadjusted age is used.

When discharged from the NICU to go home, many premature babies are behind on size, since the physical stress of prematurity affects the ability to grow. While most babies catch up in growth with their peers, what is most important is that your baby continues to follow her growth curve. *Growth is a concern anytime your baby is losing weight or dropping in the percentiles* (falling to a lower curved line on the growth curve). This should be evaluated immediately.

If you have concerns about growth, the first step is to make sure the measurements are accurate. Weight is generally accurate, but height frequently is not. When your baby is less than two years old, height is recorded lying down, when she's over age two, it's recorded standing up. To get an accurate reading with either method requires patience and a fair bit of attention to detail, because children tend to squirm and either stand on their tiptoes or slouch. Pay attention to how the height is recorded and, if possible, get the same person to measure at each visit.

Don't let anyone rush you. This is a very important piece of information. Some clinics (typically those that specialize in nutritional or hormone problems) have more accurate equipment, and the medical assistants and nurses have received more training in obtaining precise measurements. About 20 percent of children referred to specialists for short stature are actually taller than previously thought when measured with more accurate equipment.

Some premature babies may look overweight for several months, because height often lags behind weight—it's easier for the body to gain weight than to grow in length. This doesn't mean a baby is overweight, and calories should not be reduced, as this will further affect growth. Your baby will eventually grow into her weight.

Determining Catch-up Growth

Your baby's first two years are the time she has to catch up on her growth; however, there's a wide range for normal (anywhere between the 5th and the 95th percentile). To pick the most appropriate "catch-up target" for height, calculate your baby's predicted adult height.

> Formula for predicted adult height: Add the mother's height and the father's height and divide that number by two. Subtract 6.4 cm (2½ inches) from this number to calculate a girl's predicted height. For a boy, add 6.4 cm (2½ inches).

Using the growth chart for ages 2 to 20 in the Appendix, mark your child's predicted adult height in black with an ✕ on the vertical line directly below the age of 20. (Use the centimeter/inch guide immediately to the right for guidance.) Look where this ✕ falls in relation to the percentile marks (numbered 5, 10, 25, 50, 75, 90, 95) that are immediately to the right of your mark. Now mark your child's current height on the chart with an × in red (or any other color) on the vertical line beneath their age. (You can only do this calculation when your child is two years or older.) If the red × is directly on one of the curved percentile lines, follow that line with your finger up to age 20 and make another mark in red. If the × falls between two lines, do your best to follow an imaginary line between the two percentile lines up to age 20 and then mark the spot. Compare the two different color × marks on the vertical line under age 20. The black is the genetically predicted adult height, and the red × is an estimate of your child's adult height if she keeps growing at the same rate. For example, if the predicted adult height is the 40th percentile and your baby is estimated to be at the 25th percentile, she is within a percentile (one curved line on the growth chart) and on track. On the other hand, if her predicted adult height is the 75th percentile and she is estimated to be at the 10th percentile (a difference of three curved percentile lines), her growth has been much more impaired. A difference of two or more percentiles is considered significant.

The predicted adult height is only an estimate, so your baby could be 10 cm (4 inches) taller or shorter. If you don't know the father's height, you can do the calculation with just the mother's height, although it will not be as accurate.

Growth Impairment

Height percentile at the age of three is fairly predictive of adult height—additional catch-up growth after this time is unlikely, although some babies with bronchopulmonary dysplasia (BPD) may continue to catch up on missed growth until they are eight years old.

It's important to remember that there's a wide range of normal height and weight. However, children below the 5th percentile in height have short stature and those at or below the 5th percentile for weight are underweight. Children between the 6th and 10th percentile are considered at risk for being short stature or underweight. While short stature may be due to prematurity, other common causes include:

- **Difficulty meeting nutritional needs.**
- **Intrauterine growth restriction (IUGR)** (see chapter 2), which affects the way the body is programmed to grow, even before delivery. Many babies with IUGR are not capable of achieving catch-up growth.
- **Other medical conditions,** such as bronchopulmonary dysplasia or pneumonia. Illness is physically stressful. Growth hormone deficiency may also be a factor.

If nutritional intake is sufficient and other medical conditions have been excluded, and your child's height remains at or below the 3rd percentile by two to four years of age, she may be a candidate for growth hormone therapy. The 3rd percentile in height translates to a predicted adult height of 5 feet 4 inches for a boy and 4 feet 11 inches for a girl.

Growth hormone therapy should only be prescribed after careful nutritional analysis, thorough testing, and consultation with a pediatric endocrinologist. It requires an injection every single day and close monitoring of blood levels. Risks include diabetes, eye problems, and inflammation of the pancreas.

Growth hormone triggers cells to grow—it's like fertilizer. How much additional growth your child may get varies significantly. For some children, this therapy may mean several centimeters of additional height, and for others the response will be less. The gain in height you see in the first year of therapy is predictive of the ultimate response. Close management with a pediatric endocrinologist will help you make the best decisions for your child.

Nutrition

To catch up on missed growth during the third trimester, premature babies need to eat more calories per unit of body weight than full-term babies. Most premature babies are discharged needing 22 to 30 calories per 30 ml (ounce) of food, depending on their birth weight and medical conditions. Breast milk has 20 calories/30 ml, so many breast-fed babies will need additional calories. One option is to alternate breast-feeding with bottle-feeding, using a higher-calorie formula. You can also pump and add a high-calorie supplement. Human milk fortifier can be used until your baby weighs about 3,600 g (8 lbs). Other options for increasing calories in breast milk include adding any one of the following:

- **Powdered baby formula.**
- **Specially formulated additives,** such as *Microlipid, Moducal, Polycose,* or *Promod.*
- **Oils, such as safflower and coconut.** Don't worry about giving extra fat—it's the most efficient way to add additional calories.

When breast milk is unavailable there's a wide range of premature formulas to meet your baby's nutritional needs, although standard infant formulas (20 calories/30 ml) can also be mixed in such a way as to increase the calories.

The specific choice of calorie supplement or formula depends on your baby's age, weight, and underlying medical conditions. Think of high-calorie formulas and calorie supplements to breast milk as prescription medication—don't start them, change the dose, or stop them without first consulting with your baby's primary care provider and/or her registered dietician.

If you or your provider has concerns about nutrition, it's best to consult with a registered dietician who can calculate your baby's specific requirements and give you the best advice in how to meet her nutritional needs. Record everything your baby eats for several days before the visit, so the dietician can calculate her current calories, protein, and fat intake.

Weight can drop when your baby starts to eat solids, such as cereals and vegetables, because these foods are lower in calories than breast milk or formula. When you first introduce solids, limit the amount so you don't affect your baby's intake of breast milk or formula. To increase the calorie content, your doctor may recommend adding butter or even one of the powered additives (*Promod, Polycose,* etc.). A tablespoon of butter improves the taste of pureed vegetables in addition to adding 120 calories. Make sure you consult with your baby's primary care provider about when and how you should introduce solids, because the motor skills to eat safely may be delayed for a premature baby. When your baby turns one year of age, you can also supplement her diet with a high-calorie meal replacement such as *Pediasure* or *Kids Boost*, or add *Super Soluble Duocal*, an even higher-calorie powdered additive, to her food. Do not introduce cow's milk before the age of one, because unlike breast milk or formula, cow's milk isn't nutritionally complete for infants. Only after one year of age, if the rest of the diet includes a good amount of other foods that make up for the shortcomings of milk, should cow's milk be introduced.

If your baby is fed with an NG tube or a G-tube, you will use breast milk or formula as described above. When your baby turns one, she'll be switched to a specific formula for tube feeding, such as *Kindercal* or *Pediasure Enteral Formula*. Your dietician may have specific recommendations; however, the ultimate selection may depend on what's covered by your insurance company or Medicaid.

Except for my 26 weeks of pregnancy, I have been on one seemingly continuous (and rather unsuccessful) diet since the age of 16. I know the calorie count, fat grams, and fiber content of every food. I know what I'm supposed to do to lose weight (eat less and exercise more), but I just can't seem to commit for longer than a few months. Therefore, the irony that Oliver, because of his heart and lung problems, needs to eat more than I do is not entirely lost on me.

Oliver eats my dream diet. When I go for coffee, Victor gets a hot chocolate and Oliver gets a cup of whipped cream. I hide butter in his food. I ply him with bacon, cheese, avocado, and eggs. I have to prepare these meals, and I do my best not to sneak a bite of the leftovers, because everything *does* taste better with a tablespoon of butter.

When we visit the doctor and we go over his intake I can, *of course*, reel off a list of the most calorie-laden, fat-dense foods, amazing his doctors and dietician with my ability to state the nutritional content of every food by heart. I have had almost 30 years of practice. Who would have thought it would eventually pay off?

Feeding Problems

Some babies have difficulty eating. Common reasons include:

- **Fatigue.** It takes a lot of energy to eat, and some babies don't have enough to make it through a feed every three to four hours.
- **Problems with oral-motor skills,** either weakness or coordination difficulties with sucking, chewing, and swallowing.
- **Poor appetite.**
- **Oral aversion,** a sensory condition leading to food refusal.
- **Gastroesophageal reflux.** (See chapter 24.) Spitting up and vomiting mean lost calories, and if it hurts, some babies will stop eating.
- **Calorie need is too high.** Even a baby with the best appetite and good feeding skills can only eat so much.
- **Difficulties judging hunger.** Unlike the reliable signal given by term babies, crying is a relatively late sign of hunger for a premature baby.

A team approach is often required to understand the reason behind feeding difficulties and how they may be affecting growth. Medical professionals who can help assemble the pieces of the puzzle include your baby's primary care provider, an occupational therapist or speech therapist with expertise in managing feeding difficulties, a dietician, and possibly other specialists such as a gastroenterologist, a neurologist, and an endocrinologist. Many hospitals have specific feeding clinics where all the specialists work together. Interventions will depend on your baby's health and age.

Weakness in the facial muscles and oral aversion are treated with specialized occupational therapy. If appetite is an issue, a medication called *cyproheptadine* (*Periactin*) can be helpful. This is an antihistamine (allergy medication) but a side effect is increased appetite. It's very safe, although it can make some children drowsy, which can affect eating. It's hard to predict the effect, but for many babies it can lead to significant weight gain.

Victor adored his bottle. Even though he vomited out his nose after almost every feed, he was in heaven with his bottle, so I figured food would be a snap.

He tried sweet potatoes. He seemed to tolerate a few bites, but after 45 minutes the meal came out his nose and that was that. Sweet potatoes obviously hurt a lot more than formula on the way up and out, and he would not touch solid food again. He would take a bottle and put any toy in his mouth, but he gagged and turned his head at solid food. He vomited if we tried to force him.

After more than two years of occupational therapy, a dedicated home exercise program, and strategic meals with other kids, we progressed to a sippy cup and food that dissolved in his mouth—Cheetos and meringues. I tried finger painting with pudding, but Victor wiped his fingers on a towel while Oliver greedily licked his clean. It appeared as if Victor would be taking his sippy cup to college.

In my heart I felt he had the physical skills to eat. When he hadn't vomited in more than a year, I asked our pediatrician what would happen if I physically forced food into his mouth. He gave the okay.

I bought the finest quality, thinnest wafer of chocolate—something that would dissolve quickly. I picked chocolate because it not only tastes good, it triggers the release of endorphins, chemicals that make us feel good.

I offered the chocolate, and of course he refused, so I pried his mouth open, pinned his arms behind his back, and popped in the chocolate wafer, all the while saying, "Victor, that's chocolate, it's chocolate." I felt horrible.

At first he kicked and screamed, but as the chocolate melted his face relaxed and he started using his sign language. Over and over he signed, "More, more." That day he ate a whole chocolate bar. To me it was as if he had eaten a four-course meal. We started with chocolate bars at mealtime, but unlike Cheetos, chocolate can become cake, cookies, and pancakes. Finally I had a way to introduce other foods and textures.

I still feel some momentary pangs of guilt, but sometimes you just have to trust your instinct.

Babies who cannot consume enough calories and have significant growth concerns may need a feeding tube if other therapies are ineffective at increasing the calories to the required level. This may start as a naso-gastric tube, or NG tube. (See chapter 11.) Additional calories, even for a few weeks, may increase energy levels and help stimulate eating. Repeatedly inserting an NG tube (which may be necessary, as they're easily pulled out) may cause discomfort and further contribute to defensive oral behavior. Some babies will need a G-tube, or gastrostomy tube, which is a feeding tube inserted during a small surgery from the skin into the stomach. For some babies and parents, a G-tube is a better long-term solution.

A G-tube is easy to manage, and most parents become adept at changing the equipment in a very short period of time. Feeds can be given continuously throughout the day and the night, or just overnight as a supplement to what is eaten during the day. Tube feeds can increase the risk of gastroesophageal reflux, so a surgical procedure to prevent reflux, called a **fundoplication,** may also be performed. (See chapter 24.)

Oral Aversion

Oral aversion is a refusal to eat, and it's more common among babies who were tube-fed for more than three weeks. Oral aversion is a sensory processing disorder in which food produces an abnormal sensation. For some babies it's all foods, and for other it may be liquids, solids, or even a particular texture. Some babies and children with oral aversion drool excessively because they're unaware of what's going on with their mouths. These sensory problems may also lead to overstuffing the mouth with food. Other babies with oral aversion refuse to put anything in their mouths, while some will put toys in their mouth, but not food.

Oral aversion may make feeding a challenge from the start or may appear when your baby tries new foods. Overcoming oral aversion is a slow process. Here are a few ways to help:

- **Encourage pacifier use.** Sucking strengthens the muscles and helps to stimulate the gastrointestinal tract.
- **Offer appropriate toys to mouth.** The more your baby is able to put inside her mouth, the more stimulation she will learn to process.
- **Work with an experienced speech or occupational therapist (OT).** Both you and your child need to connect with her therapist. If you don't see at least some minor progress after several months, consider an opinion from another therapist.
- **Home exercises.** Your OT will prescribe home exercises. She may also recommend therapy tools that vibrate and have different textures as well as special feeding equipment. Blowing soap bubbles through rings can help strengthen muscles and introduces some fun into the routine. If you keep the bubbles for oral therapy time only, it may help to keep your baby interested. They are hard for most kids to resist.
- **Time.** Many children increase their tolerance of foods once they begin to develop the motor skills to feed themselves finger foods. In addition, the peer pressure of watching other children eat can be very beneficial.
- **Do not get into battles.** Children are looking for ways to exert independence, especially as they begin to realize the power of saying no. Even babies learn quickly that food refusal is an effective weapon. Keep your stress level down. Your baby will pick up on your cues, and it will be harder to get her to eat. Take three deep breaths before every meal and any time you feel yourself getting worked up.
- **Establish meal rituals.** Your child might not want to eat or even be able to eat, but include her in the social aspect of eating (although keep in mind that a toddler might only manage five minutes). Do what you can to make mealtime fun. Discourage wandering around with food. If she will eat at least one food, make sure it's on her plate so she participates in the meal.

- **If appropriate, take advantage of inpatient feeding programs,** which are intensive programs that involve many experienced specialists.

It's important to remember that a mouthful or a small bite, or even the willingness to put a new toy in the mouth, is a sign of progress. Keep a journal, and remember it may take months and months before you notice any real change. Learning to eat for a child with an oral aversion is a frustrating process of slow and gradual desensitization, but with time every baby who has the physical ability to eat will eventually do so.

24

The Preemie Gastrointestinal Tract: Constipation, Reflux, Food Allergies, and Colic

Gastrointestinal problems are common, especially in the first few years at home. While there are generally no quick fixes, there are treatment options. As with many of the consequences of prematurity, improvement comes with a combination of time and persistence with therapies.

Constipation

Constipation is the infrequent passage of stools, painful and hard stools, or straining during bowel movements. The normal frequency of stooling varies significantly with age and diet. When bowel movements become less frequent, the stool increases in size and become hard and dry. Passing large, hard, dry stool is painful and physically difficult.

Some grunting and straining during bowel movements is normal, but it's abnormal if your baby (less than one year adjusted) takes more than 10 minutes to pass a stool. Toddlers and older children may also strain, but withholding stool is more common. Withholding is tightening the pelvic muscles to prevent passing a potentially painful bowel movement.

Typically a child will get red in the face, stiffen up, stand on her tiptoes, or rock back and forth. It might look as if she is straining to pass a stool, but she's doing the exact opposite. It's frightening and painful to have a large bowel movement, and the reaction to try to prevent it is understandable; however, withholding creates larger bowel movements, because the stool starts to accumulate in the rectum. These larger stools become even harder and more difficult to pass, perpetuating the cycle. In some cases, the stools get large enough that fecal material may leak out around the retained stool. Older children may also complain of belly pain and their appetite may decrease.

Constipation is uncommon if your baby is consuming only breast milk. It's such a well-designed food that very little material remains in the bowel after digestion. Bowel movements are also typically soft, which makes them easy to pass. Some breast-fed babies have frequent smaller movements throughout the day, but it's not unusual for stool to accumulate and pass every four to five days. If a breast-fed baby is not straining, uncomfortable, or irritable, it's fine to go seven days between bowel movements.

Infant formulas are not absorbed as well, so there's more stool. This can lead to constipation, because it's difficult for the intestines to handle this extra bulk. Soy formula tends to produce even more constipation than cow's milk formula. A formula-fed infant under the age of one typically has one to two bowel movements a day.

When cereal is introduced, the added bulk may slow the bowels even more. Adding vegetables and fruit improves constipation, because the fiber in these foods draws water into the bowel, which helps to keep the stool soft and move things along. By the age of one most babies have one to two bowel movements a day. However, some have more and some have less. If the bowel movements are not hard and pass easily, then there is little cause for concern.

While diet plays an important role, many premature babies have additional factors that influence the bowel and contribute to constipation, such as:

- **Weaker muscles and coordination problems,** which make it difficult to physically push out stool while simultaneously relaxing the muscles around the rectum.
- **Slower bowels,** from illness, stress, and medications. Medical conditions that can cause constipation include an underactive thyroid, cerebral palsy, cystic fibrosis, and Hirschsprung's disease (reduced or absent in the bowel).
- **Inadequate fiber intake** for children who are eating solids. This may be due to food selection, oral aversions that limit choices, or the need to preferentially offer higher-calorie foods (because fats and protein have no fiber). There are no specific recommendations for fiber intake for children less than three years of age, but children ages three to 18 should eat enough grams of fiber each day to equal their age plus five. (For example, a six-year-old should eat 11 grams of fiber per day.)
- **Sensory issues with toileting.** Some children have difficulty with the feel of the toilet seat or the sensation of passing a bowel movement. This may contribute to withholding behavior.

Treatment for constipation depends on your baby's age and the contributing factors. Always discuss any treatments you plan to start at home with your baby's provider *before* starting. For babies less than one year old (adjusted), treatment options include:

- **Karo corn syrup,** 1 to 2 tsp per bottle.
- **Barley malt extract,** 2 to 10 ml/240 ml of milk or juice. (It smells.)
- **Sorbitol-containing fruits and fruit juices,** specifically prunes, pears, apricots, and apples. Fruit is a better option than juice. It contains fiber, so it is more effective. In addition, if your baby has reflux, the acidic juice may be irritating. Fruit juice also has very limited nutritional value and the volume and calories decrease your baby's appetite, preventing her from eating nutritionally complete foods.

- **Glycerin suppositories** are safe at any age. Infant suppositories are available, but may need to be cut lengthwise to fit.

Additional treatments for older children include:

- **Fiber supplements** if your child is three years or older and her fiber intake is low. Discuss the appropriate dose with your child's primary care provider or gastroenterologist. Choose a supplement that dissolves well, like *Benefiber*. The stool will be larger, so be prepared for larger, more painful bowel movements initially. Once stooling is more frequent, size will be less of an issue.
- **Polyethylene glycol powder,** or *Miralax,* which is an over-the-counter laxative that can be mixed with food or fluids. *Miralax* isn't absorbed by the body and is a safe long-term option. The dose varies depending on your baby's age and size and should only be started after talking with your baby's primary care provider or gastroenterologist.
- **Other laxatives,** which should only be used under close medical supervision. Non-stimulant laxatives, like *milk of magnesia, lactulose,* and *sorbitol,* are preferred. These medications work in the same way as *Karo syrup, barley extract,* and *Miralax,* by drawing water into the bowel. Stimulant laxatives, such as *docusate* (*Dulcolax*) and *senna* (*Senokot*), make the bowel contract more forcefully. They're more likely to cause painful cramping and should only be used if specifically recommended by your baby's doctor, when your baby is over the age of one, and other options have failed.
- **Mineral oil,** a lubricant that makes it easier for the bowel to move food along. While it's natural and not absorbed by the body, even a few drops in the lungs can cause severe problems. It should never be used for babies less than one year old or at any age if your child has reflux.

If your baby is voluntarily withholding stool, it's important to recognize and treat it. Options include:

- **Regular use of laxatives** to keep the stool loose, making the physical act of withholding difficult. Once your baby has had several looser, non-painful bowel movements, the reflex to withhold may lessen; however, it may take a while to unlearn this pattern of abnormal stooling.
- **Sitting your child on the toilet after meals,** because eating stimulates the bowels to move, and this is the easiest time to have a bowel movement.
- **Biofeedback,** in which a trained practitioner works with your child so she learns to have better control of the muscles needed to stool. Special equipment is involved.

Persistent constipation despite appropriate therapy increases the chance your baby could have another underlying condition. Testing may be necessary, including:

- **A sweat chloride test,** which is the test for cystic fibrosis. This is a painless test that evaluates the level of chloride in your baby's sweat.
- **A thyroid screen,** especially if your baby was stooling well but has now become constipated. Testing is not needed if your baby is less than a year old, as she was tested at birth.
- **Evaluation for cerebral palsy,** which is a muscle condition (see chapter 25) that produces abnormal movement. It can affect how the bowels function. A pediatric specialist, typically a neurologist or physiatrist, will evaluate your baby for cerebral palsy.

Reflux

The backward movement of stomach acid and food from the stomach into the esophagus, called reflux (see chapter 12), can be a persistent problem after coming home. Common reasons that reflux persists:

- **Muscle weakness,** which is especially common in the first year for premature babies. The lower esophageal sphincter (the muscle that separates the esophagus from the stomach) will be affected just like any other muscle. The strength and coordination of the lower esophageal sphincter will improve with time.

- **Cerebral palsy,** which can cause coordination problems with eating that increase air swallowing. The lower esophageal sphincter may also not work effectively and the stomach and bowels may be slower, so food sits in the stomach for a longer time.
- **Calorie density of meals.** Many premature babies and children need more calories; however, calorie-rich foods slow stomach-emptying and may contribute to reflux by leaving stomach contents available to be refluxed.
- **Other medical conditions,** such as breathing problems or infection.
- **Exposure to cigarette smoke,** which decreases the strength of the lower esophageal sphincter. Smoke exposure also triggers coughing, which increases abdominal pressure, also causing reflux.
- **Medications that may affect alertness.**

Many premature babies are diagnosed with reflux while in the hospital. (See chapter 12.) As your baby gets older, additional symptoms or reflux-related complications may appear, such as:

- **Sleeping problems,** because reflux is often worse at night. Not only is your baby lying down for an extended period, but all our muscles are weaker when we are tired.
- **Chronic cough, congestion, snoring, or hoarse voice.** Over time the acidity of the refluxed stomach contents irritates and causes swelling in the throat, sinuses, and nasal passages.
- **Torticollis,** which is an abnormal tightening in the muscles on one side of the neck. (See chapter 26.) Pain from reflux may cause your baby to constantly turn her head in one direction, which can tighten the neck muscle on the affected side.
- **Taking longer to eat or refusal to eat,** which may be a sign that eating is painful due to inflammation in the esophagus or stomach.

- **Difficulty gaining weight or weight loss.**
- **Blood in vomit,** a sign of bleeding from an inflamed esophagus. If this happens, you should call your baby's provider immediately.
- **Pneumonia,** due to food and stomach contents passing into the lungs. Reflux-related pneumonia is more common in the right lung.

The treatment options for reflux are the same at home as in the hospital. (See chapter 12 for medication options.) Limit time in the car seat, because this position causes increased pressure on your baby's stomach, which facilitates reflux. Sleeping on the stomach is not recommended due to sudden infant death syndrome (SIDS). Elevating the head of the crib can help, though a significant elevation can cause your baby to slide down on her mattress. A Tucker sling, which is a harness system made of fabric, can keep your baby at a 30-degree angle, which can be helpful for some babies. A Tucker sling can be purchased online (some insurance companies will reimburse you) or borrowed from a friend, or if you or someone you know can sew, you can make your own version.

Try thickening feeds with *SimplyThick* or baby cereal (oatmeal or rice) if your baby is taking a bottle. If she's taking solids, keep her diet bland with cereals, toast, rice, bananas, plain pasta, and Cheerios. Avoid citrus fruits and juices, tomato-based foods, and fried and other high-fat foods.

Even if acid-blocker medications such as H2 blockers and proton pump inhibitors (see chapter 12) were ineffective while your baby was in the hospital, they may be worth trying again if symptoms persist or get worse at home. While acid-blockers don't stop the reflux, they slow the production of acid so that the refluxed material is less acidic, allowing the esophagus to heal itself.

Important considerations for acid-blockers include:

- **The easiest H2 blocker to administer is** *ranitidine.* The liquid is generic, but it does contain alcohol, which could be irritating to an inflamed stomach. *Ranitidine* also comes as an effervescent tablet, which can be dissolved in water and may be less irritating. *Ranitidine* is a good drug, but it may not suppress enough acid for some babies. If symptoms persist after two to three weeks, talk with your doctor about another option.

- *Ranitidine* **may become less effective over time.** If your baby was doing well on *ranitidine* but then she worsens, switching to a proton pump inhibitor (PPI) may help.

- **A proton pump inhibitor, if needed, should be baby friendly.** *Zegrid* and *Prevacid* are the easiest options for a baby or young child. *Zegrid* (*omeprazole*) is a powder that you mix with water and syringe into your baby's mouth. *Prevacid* (*lanoseprazole*) is available as a dissolvable tablet (hold the tablet against the inside of your baby's cheek for a few minutes and it will dissolve). Don't use over-the-counter *Prilosec* (a brand of *omeprazole*) if your child cannot swallow pills, as these tablets must not be split. Other PPIs are available, including *Nexium* (*esomeprazole*), *Protonix* (*pantoprazole*), and *Aciphex* (*rabeprazole*); however, a pharmacist must compound them into a liquid and they are only stable for 14 days. If you've been getting a 30-day supply and symptoms return a week or two before you're due for a refill, ask for a 14-day supply at a time or a PPI that does not require compounding.

- **The contents of PPI capsules should not be crushed or chewed.** When your baby can eat food from a spoon, open the capsules and sprinkle the beads on soft food, such as cottage cheese or pudding. Make sure it is a food that allows her to swallow the beads whole.

The PPIs on the market are all very effective. If symptoms have not improved after two to four weeks, either the dose is not right or your baby's symptoms are not acid related. Switching to another PPI is common practice; however, it is unlikely to make that much difference. *Metoclopramide* (*Reglan*) may be considered if there are persistent reflux symptoms, frequent regurgitation, and delayed stomach-emptying.

When conservative measures and medication are not enough to control symptoms or your baby is losing weight, has apneic spells, or develops pneumonia, testing may be necessary. Tests may include:

- **An upper GI series,** to rule out a hiatal hernia. (See chapter 12.)
- **An endoscopy,** in which a gastroenterologist looks at the esophagus and stomach with a telescope placed through the mouth. This test identifies physical abnormalities that could be contributing to reflux as well as inflammation and ulcers. Several biopsies (small pinches of tissue) will be taken and sent to the lab for further tests. The tissue can also be tested for the *H. pylori* bacteria. Biopsies may indicate inflammation not seen with the naked eye. A general anesthetic is needed for an endoscopy.
- **A pH study,** which is a test to see how often acid is refluxing backward into the esophagus. It requires a nasogastric tube with a special monitor that continuously records the pH (acid level) in the lower portion of the esophagus. The tube can be uncomfortable for some babies. A pH study is often combined with an endoscopy, so the tube is placed while your baby is still asleep. The test is typically performed over 24 hours, and while the monitor records the acidity, you record your baby's symptoms. If acid reflux matches the symptoms, then the two are related.

Babies with serious complications, such as pneumonia, weight loss, apnea related to vomiting, or ulcers of the esophagus or stomach despite maximal medical therapy, may need surgery. The procedure is called a Nissen fundoplication, which involves wrapping some of the stomach around the esophagus. This tightens the opening where the esophagus enters the stomach, allowing food to go in but preventing it from going back up.

A Nissen fundoplication is major abdominal surgery, although it's typically performed with an operating telescope, so the scars are tiny and the recovery fairly quick. Some babies and children have difficulty eating after a Nissen and may need a **gastrostomy tube** (a tube surgically placed through the belly wall into the stomach) to receive nutrition. The G-tube can contribute to problems with food refusal and oral aversions (see chapters 11 and 23), and many babies will need intensive occupational therapy to start eating. However, for babies and children with severe reflux, the benefits of the surgery outweigh these potential risks.

Victor's reflux and vomiting did not improve with *ranitidine*, two different PPIs, *metoclopramide*, and thickened feeds. To keep him from vomiting there were many nights he needed to sleep with me, upright in a chair. We were referred to a pediatric gastroenterologist.

Three tests were recommended. As a doctor, I know tests are generally only indicated when the results will change treatment. So I thought a lot about how each test might affect Victor's care. For a test to be useful, it would have to tell me whether surgery was indicated for his reflux.

He had the barium swallow. It was very stressful, because he wouldn't drink the barium. He was held down while it was syringed into his mouth, and we both cried. However, he didn't have a hiatal hernia. If he had, surgery would have been the answer.

Then the endoscopy was performed. I almost had a panic attack as he went off to sleep. However, if he had severe inflammation and an ulcer despite maximal medical therapy, then I would consider surgery. It would also be helpful to know if the anatomy of his esophagus and stomach was normal. Everything was fine.

Much to the specialist's surprise, I refused the pH probe. Victor vomited more than 10 times a day, so I didn't need a test to tell me he had reflux. It didn't matter to me if he refluxed 10 or a 100 times a day, because he was only unhappy when he vomited. The amount of reflux would not influence my decision for surgery, only complications would.

I'm probably biased. As a pain medicine specialist, I treat a lot of people who have surgical complications. No one expects to have problems after surgery, but it's a real risk. So as long as his medical health was not suffering, I figured we would just try to wait it out. There are worse things than sleeping in a chair.

Food Allergies

A food allergy is a reaction to the protein in food that causes local inflammation in the gastrointestinal tract. It can cause the body's immune system to behave inappropriately and trigger asthma and skin problems like eczema. (See chapter 26.) The inflammation in the GI tract can involve the esophagus, the stomach, and the intestines, producing symptoms such as pain, feeding problems, and difficulty gaining weight. On the surface it can be very difficult to distinguish reflux from food allergies. Symptoms that are seen with food allergies and not reflux include diarrhea, which is the result of inflammation and spasm in the intestines; blood in the stool; and eczema.

The most common allergy is to cow's milk proteins, although 50 percent of children who are allergic to cow's milk are also allergic to soy. Allergies to eggs, nuts, and shellfish can also occur.

Formulas for premature babies use cow's milk protein, so formula-fed babies are at greatest risk. While food allergies are much less common among breast-fed babies (because the way a mother's body processes the proteins is protective), proteins in mom's diet can sometimes be a trigger. A food allergy can also develop later when you introduce these foods into your child's diet.

The best way to see if a food allergy is playing a role in your baby's symptoms is to eliminate the food from her diet. Start by eliminating cow's milk and soy, as these are the two most likely offenders. It may take four to six weeks for the inflammation in the gastrointestinal tract to settle down, so you need to try the changes for six weeks. Always consult with your baby's provider before making any dietary changes.

If you're breast-feeding, eliminate milk and soy-based products from your diet. This includes other foods such as chocolate, margarine, and non-dairy creamer, as milk proteins may be used in the manufacturing of all these products. You can consider eliminating eggs, nuts, and shellfish, too, if eliminating cow's milk and soy is not helpful.

If your baby is formula-fed, switching to a hypoallergenic or "predigested" formula may help with a food allergy. (See Table 1.) Proteins are composed of long chains of building blocks called amino acids. In hypoallergenic formulas, the protein chains are broken down into shorter lengths and therefore are less likely to trigger an allergic reaction. Partially hydrolyzed formulas are partially broken down and still have some longer protein chains, while hydrolyzed formulas are all shorter chains. Amino acid (also called elemental) formulas are made from the amino acid building blocks and contain no protein chains. They are the least likely to trigger an allergic response and are easiest for the bowel to digest. A partially

TABLE 1: Formulas for Cow's Milk Allergy

Formula Options	Formula
Partially hydrolyzed	Nestlé Good Start Enfamil Gentlease
Hydrolyzed	Nutramigen Alimentum Pregestemil
Amino acid	Neocate Neocate-1-plus* Nutramigen AA EleCare Vivonex*

*For children age one and older

hydrolyzed or hydrolyzed formula will treat most allergies, but some babies need an amino acid formula. Don't use a soy formula, as it can trigger food allergies and is low in many nutrients important for a premature baby.

Before switching your baby's formula, talk with her primary care provider, gastroenterologist, or allergist. These formulas are also more expensive. (The greater the degree of protein breakdown, the more expensive they are.) You may be able to get one of these formulas through your insurance or through WIC, if you're eligible. You can also check eBay—you'll be surprised what you find and the price is often much better.

Many babies will not eat pre-digested formulas because they have a foul smell and taste terrible, although adding some flavored syrup, a sugar substitute, like NutraSweet, or a drop of vanilla extract can help. Ask a registered dietician for tips and tricks to make these formulas more palatable.

Tests that may help in the decision-making process, include:

- **Testing the stool for blood.** This is an easy, painless test, done in the office, that may be performed if a food allergy is suspected. If blood is present, the cause may be inflammation—possibly from a food allergy, but it could also be from something else. A negative test does not rule out a food allergy.

- **Colonoscopy,** which is a procedure in which a specialist looks in the intestines (with a special telescope) for inflammation or other problems. Inflammation is not always visible to the eye, so biopsies will be taken and evaluated under the microscope.

Blood tests to look for antibodies, the substance in the blood that is interacting with the food protein, are seldom helpful unless your baby or child has a reaction to food that includes hives, eczema, or difficulty breathing.

Some parents and providers feel comfortable switching formula with out tests, because ultimately what matters is solving the problem. If you try a new formula and it works, the actual reason is far less important. The good news is that for most children, milk protein allergy goes away with time. Talk with your baby's doctor about when you can switch formulas or reintroduce certain foods into your diet or your baby's diet.

Colic

Colic is the term for excessive fussiness and crying, which is crying for more than three hours a day, three days a week, for three weeks. Gastrointestinal problems can play a role in this irritability, so it's important to seriously consider constipation, reflux, and food allergies as the cause. If after a thorough evaluation no contributing factor is identified, it's possible that colic may be a sign of any one of the following:

- **Fatigue.** This may explain why irritability is worse at the end of the day. Premature babies tend to have more disorganized sleep patterns and expend a lot of energy eating and breathing. In addition, many babies are drained by illness, physical challenges, and daily physical and occupational therapy. If you're exhausted, your baby is probably more exhausted.

- **An immature nervous system** that is erroneously amplifying or misinterpreting input from the outside world. (See chapter 8.) The bowels are at significant risk because they have more nerves than any other part of the body, including the brain. In addition, the bowels are constantly functioning, so there's no time for rest and recovery. Some doctors, like Harvey Karp, MD (author of *The Happiest Baby on the Block*), have coined the term "the fourth trimester" to explain this time needed for the nervous system to adapt to its new environment. Many premature babies (and their parents) experience an extended fourth trimester.

A month after coming home, Oliver developed colic. He was the happiest baby during the day. He ate without difficulty, slept well, and never fussed. However, at 7 PM Dr. Jekyll became Mr. Hyde. He would cry inconsolably until 11 PM, when the storm simply rolled out of town.

Hypoallergenic formulas and reflux medications did nothing. Tony drove him around in the car, but he cried. We tried placing him in the car seat on the dryer, but he still cried. Swings and bouncy chairs brought no reprieve, and neither did simethicone anti-gas drops or increasing his oxygen levels. The only solution was to walk in a circle at a particular pace.

I didn't think it was fatigue—the time he cried did not vary based on his activity. It was always 7 PM. We could practically set our watch by it. It was this witching hour that led me to believe that his nervous system was involved and this was a fourth-trimester issue.

Our bodies have diurnal rhythms—meaning chemical messengers are released at specific times during the day and night. This intricate autopilot sequencing allows optimal interaction with our environment. I theorized Oliver's system was misaligned—like a malfunction in the autotimer for a porch light.

So the only answer was walking in circles. Even with all we had been through, Oliver's colic was one of the hardest things in our first year at home. It's terrible and cruelly disempowering when you know your baby is in distress and all you can do is bide your time. Venting with other parents who had been there helped the most. They all reassured us it would stop, but secretly we didn't believe them, and Tony was resigned to walking in circles for the next year.

And then one night, about three months later, he just stopped crying.

25

<hr>

Milestones and
Neurological Concerns

Prematurity is the number one cause of disability for children. While it's not possible to repair damage to the nervous system, early recognition of delays and impairments with appropriate interventions will offer the best prognosis for your child. The nervous system is most plastic in the first few years of life and therefore has an amazing capacity to adapt and rewire itself.

Motor Milestones

Motor development follows a predictable sequence, starting from the head and progressing downward. A fatty material called myelin insulates the nerves that control muscles. This insulation is essential in transmitting messages from the brain to produce coordinated movements of the muscles. Production of myelin begins shortly after birth, with shorter nerves completed first. So coordination of facial muscles (smiling), which are innervated by the shortest nerves, is the first motor milestone, followed by control of the neck, the trunk (ability to sit), the arms (reaching for objects), the fingers (grasping), and then legs (crawling, standing, and finally walking). Your baby's motor skills should be assessed on a regular basis to monitor development of the nervous system. (See Table 1.)

For the first two years, your baby's adjusted age should be used when assessing motor skills.

There are different motor milestones for gross and fine motor skills. Gross motor skills involve using large groups of muscles to do activities like sitting, standing, and running. Fine motor skills involve the hands for activities such as eating, getting dressed, and writing.

Premature babies are at greater risk for motor delays. A delay of 25 percent is considered significant. (For example, a baby who is 24 months adjusted age who has not met the 18-month milestones has a 25 percent delay.) In addition to milestones, it's important to be observant for other potential signs of developmental problems, including:

- **Toe walking.** Walking on tiptoes occasionally is normal, but it signals a problem when it happens most of the time.
- **Using one side of the body preferentially.** Asymmetry is not normal. Your baby should use both arms and legs equally, and they should have similar positions at rest. By the age of three your child may start to indicate a hand preference.
- **Abnormal postures,** such as keeping one arm bent at the elbow or a fist clenched.
- **Muscle tone that is either too floppy (hypotonia) or too stiff (hypertonia).**

There are several reasons for motor delays, abnormal posture, and abnormal tone, including cerebral palsy, sensory processing disorders, and autism. However, keep in mind that sometimes a motor delay is just due to prematurity and not a symptom of another disorder.

Regardless of the cause, if there are any concerns, further evaluation and intervention are necessary to improve function. Motor delays should be treated with skilled physical and occupational therapy involving exercises that strengthen muscles, develop coordination, and work on balance. Specific exercises will vary depending on the situation. Some helpful activities with specific aims:

TABLE 1: Motor Milestones

Age	Gross motor	Fine motor
At 3 months	Lifts head and chest when lying on stomach, stretches legs and kicks while lying on stomach, brings hand to mouth	Follows moving objects/person with eyes, loosely grasps objects
At 7 months	Sits unsupported, good head control, reaches for toys, rolls over both ways, supports whole weight on legs	Passes toys from one hand to the other, mouths objects, plays with toes
At 12 months	Can get into sitting position independently, crawls on belly, pulls to a stand, walks with help	Picks up small objects with thumb and forefinger, begins to use spoon, bangs two objects together, puts objects in and takes them out of container
At 18 months	Likes to push and pull things, walks up stairs with one hand held	Scribbles, stacks 2 blocks
At 24 months	Walks alone, beginning to run, walks up stairs with help, climbs up and down furniture	Feeds self with spoon, builds a tower of 3 to 4 blocks, tosses a ball
At 3 years	Rides tricycle, runs, takes stairs alternating feet, bends over without falling	Builds a tower of more than 6 blocks, draws lines with crayons, unscrews jar lids, turns pages one at a time
By 4 years	Hops and stands on one foot for 5 seconds, goes up and down stairs without help, kicks ball, throws overhand	Draws person with 2 to 4 body parts, uses scissors, draws circles and squares, copies some capital letters
By 5 years	Stands on one foot for 10 seconds, hops, swings, climbs	Draws person with body, prints some letters, dresses and undresses without help, can take care of own toilet needs

- **Use both sides of the body,** such as passing an object from one hand to another or catching a ball. Threading beads or penne pasta on a string is a great activity for older children. Using both sides of the body engages both sides of the brain, which helps to build important nervous system connections.
- **Strengthen hand muscles,** such as interlocking blocks (Duplo blocks for younger children and Lego for older), Play-Doh, and clay.
- **Improve hand-eye coordination,** such as lacing boards and pegs.
- **Strengthen mouth muscles**, such as blowing bubbles and blowing into whistles.
- **Work on thumb and finger pinching,** such as picking up dried beans. Older children can try using tweezers to pick up objects.
- **Work on balance,** such as sitting on a ball.
- **Improve arm strength,** such as holding weighted beanbags for younger children and playing wheelbarrow for older children.

Cerebral Palsy

Cerebral palsy (CP) is a condition of abnormal movement. It affects balance and posture and is caused by injury to the area of the brain that controls muscle movements. Conditions that may be involved in the development of CP include intraventricular hemorrhage (IVH) and periventricular leukomalacia (PVL, see chapter 8) as well as infection and low oxygen levels.

How a child is affected depends on the specific area of the brain that's injured. Some children have mild CP, which may appear as clumsiness, and others are severely affected, unable to walk or talk due to stiffness and abnormal movements.

CP is classified by the number of limbs involved and the character of the movements. There are four main types:

- **Spastic,** characterized by stiff, difficult movements. The stiffness is present during sleep as well as while awake.

- **Dyskinetic,** characterized by involuntary movements that may be rapid, jerky, or writhing, and **dystonia,** which appears as abnormal positions. These movements and positions may become more pronounced with stress and fatigue and go away during sleep. The arms, head, and mouth tend to be more affected than the legs.
- **Ataxic,** characterized by coordination and balance difficulties such as trouble keeping limbs and the trunk steady and abnormal eye movements.
- **Mixed,** which is a combination of some or all of the above.

The actual type of CP is less important than understanding the degree of impairment, although having a specific diagnosis may be helpful for insurance purposes when justifying services and special equipment. It may also help in explaining and understanding specific behaviors.

Cerebral palsy doesn't mean that your child will be mentally delayed—many children with CP have normal or above normal intelligence. However, the same injury that damaged the part of the brain that controls muscle movements may have caused damage to other areas of the brain as well. Children with CP are more likely to have neurological problems, such as seizures and intellectual delays, than premature children who do not have CP.

CP may be diagnosed as early as six months, but many state agencies will not accept the diagnosis until two years of age. Potential signs of CP include:

- **Delays in motor milestones.**
- **Toe walking.**
- **Persistent primitive reflexes.** A primitive reflex is a response involving the nervous system and muscles that is out of conscious control. One example is sneezing. When the nasal passages are irritated, a sneeze clears out pollens and dirt, preventing them from entering the airways and lungs where they cause damage. While some primitive reflexes, like sneezing or yawning, stay for life, most disappear in a predictable fashion as gross and fine motor skills

develop. Most primitive reflexes should disappear by 12 months adjusted age.

- **Abnormal muscle tone,** either too floppy or too stiff. Some children look like they're making scissor motions with their legs because of stiffness. A physical therapist or doctor unfamiliar with CP might confuse muscle stiffness in a baby or toddler with the ability to control muscle movements and fail to recognize that there is a problem.
- **Asymmetry in posture and movement,** including a hand preference before the age of one.
- **Persistent difficulty feeding** due to trouble coordinating sucking and swallowing.
- **Clumsiness with fine motor tasks.**

If there's any question about whether your child has CP, a referral to a specialist is advised (typically a pediatric neurologist or a pediatric physical medicine and rehabilitation physician). A specialist will make the diagnosis after a careful physical exam; however, a CT scan or MRI of the brain may be needed to rule out other conditions. Specialists will also prescribe therapy and adaptive equipment and can provide invaluable insight about community resources.

CP cannot be cured. The goal of treatment is to improve function by strengthening muscles and developing new nervous system connections. CP does not get worse; however, muscles that are in spasm can become shortened (this is called a **contracture**), which may restrict abilities. The more common therapies for CP include:

- **Physical, occupational, and speech therapy,** to strengthen muscles, build new pathways, and prevent contractures.
- **Braces to help correct abnormal postures** and prevent contractures.
- **Hippotherapy** (horseback riding), which is good for trunk control and balance.

- **Adaptive devices to improve mobility,** such as walkers and wheelchairs.
- **Injections of Botox or phenol into muscles to reduce spasm.**

My experience as a doctor told me Victor had CP when he was six months old. From then on, I would gently correct his abnormally clenched hands and his posture whenever possible. My theory: Correcting postures early on would decrease abnormal input to the brain.

Guided by an amazing physical therapist, Victor became more tolerant of stimulation, and we added new therapies every week. Tony built a table so Victor had support to stand. And no matter how hard it was, we watched him try and fail at tasks.

As he grew, I supplemented formal occupational therapy with arts and crafts and cooking. There is a fine motor skill in every craft (and pouring liquids and adding chocolate chips is just a lot more fun).

When a task was too hard, like putting on socks, I broke it down into as many small sequences as possible, making sure the first task was the easiest, because I wanted him to build confidence. So, the first step in putting on socks was opening the sock drawer, the second was picking out the socks, and so on.

When Victor still couldn't jump at the age of three, we bought a small, inflatable bouncy house where he spent hours. The extra lift helped get him off the ground with both feet. At night, Victor lay on his back and pushed against my chest with his feet, as if he were doing leg presses. I could feel where he was pressing and where he wasn't and could help coordinate the movements. It was like upside-down jumping, with balance taken out of the equation.

Somewhere along the way, Victor took over. He practices for hours to be "like the other kids." He's still a mass of primitive reflexes and shouldn't be able to do a lot of what he does, but his determination is humbling. Telling that boy he can't do something is like throwing down a dare. And that attitude has proven to be his most useful skill of all.

Sensory Processing Disorder

Sensory processing disorder, or SPD (also called **sensory integration disorder**), is a condition in which the nervous system does not process sensory input appropriately. It may involve one or more senses (touch, taste, smell, sound, or sight) or be very specific, such as an aversion to the sensation of being wet or the feel of the toilet seat.

Sensory input guides movement and behavior. We integrate feedback from all of our senses to walk, jump, eat, and even to sit quietly. With SPD, it's as if the volume control for a particular sense is wired incorrectly, resulting in far too much input or not enough. Inaccurate input about touch and balance can lead to clumsiness and motor delays, problems processing tastes and smells can contribute to oral aversions, and difficulties processing words or sounds can lead to language delays. Some sensory experiences may be perceived as unpleasant or even frightening, and a child's reactions can be incorrectly perceived as behavior problems.

SPD is more common among premature babies because the nervous system is exposed to sensory input before it's ready. SPD doesn't affect intelligence, and it doesn't mean that a child has autism; however, some children with autism have SPD, so all children with SPD should be screened for autism. Because premature babies have a higher risk of visual problems and deafness, vision and hearing should be tested before making the diagnosis of SPD.

The primary treatment for SPD is occupational therapy and home exercises. Some children may also need physical therapy and speech therapy. Treatments include:

- **Desensitization,** which is gradually introducing sensory challenges in small increments.
- **Working on transitions,** because preparing for what comes next can be helpful.
- **Working on what your child** *can* **do,** because success builds confidence and any stimulation that doesn't elicit an inappropriate response is positive.

- **Practicing activities that require balance,** because this involves a lot of sensory feedback.
- **Adaptive devices that make activities more tolerable.** One example is a weighted blanket or vest, as some children with SPD find deep pressure comforting.
- **Strengthening weak muscles** and other therapies for motor delays.
- **Exposure to peers** in play therapy. Children have a strong desire to fit in, so by watching other children, they can model the desired behavior. However, some children find the stimulation of groups too challenging.

Oliver and Victor are opposites on the sensory spectrum. Oliver has sensory neglect and is completely unaware (and doesn't care) when he's drenched in mud, while a drop of food on Victor's clothes used to cause what can only be called a "freakout."

First, off would come his soiled shirt, and he would change clothes. Still crying as he continued to eat, his tremors would increase, so he'd spill again. Off came the next shirt, and more hysterics ensued. Over and over the cycle repeated itself, gathering force, until he had spilled five or six times, everyone was hysterical, and no acceptable shirts were left. Because Victor can *only* wear blue polo shirts and button-down shirts, he could easily go through his week's supply of young Republican attire before he was halfway through a meal.

I was okay with his clothes issues. He can go through life only wearing polo shirts and fit in just fine. However, he had to learn to accept a spill or two, especially with his tremor.

The first meal with the "no change rule" involved a lot of screaming, but we didn't waver. I prepared as many spillproof meals as his oral aversion would allow and sometimes I fed him, because getting him through a meal without a complete meltdown seemed to tune down the volume on hysterics the next time he spilled. Crying and screaming were fuel for his sensory fire.

It was hard and took the better part of a year, but we got there. We didn't eat out at all, because my kids enjoy an audience. Victor now "motor plans" each bite to avoid a spill, but it still happens from time to time. I can see him tense. I know it bothers him, and there may even be an occasional tear, but then he pulls himself together and gets on with the task at hand. Oliver, on the other hand, is still struggling with the concept of wiping his face, so he fits in with the others boys just fine.

Managing sensory issues can become more challenging with time, because being oppositional is a normal part of childhood. As children grow, they're looking for opportunities to say "no" and "I don't like that." Instinct is a good guide—with time you may learn physical cues that help distinguish between *cannot* and *will not*. Because children are testing boundaries, it's important to pick your battles and focus your energy on correcting behaviors that are likely to have the greatest negative impact. For example, learning to sit on a toilet seat is more important than wearing a shirt with buttons.

Autism Spectrum Disorders

Children with autism spectrum disorders (ASD) have difficulties with social development. Several conditions are part of the autism spectrum, but the most common are:

- Autism
- Asperger's Syndrome
- Pervasive Developmental Disorder-Not Otherwise Specified (PDD-NOS)

It's unknown if the conditions in the autism spectrum represent distinct medical problems with similarities or if they represent different expressions of the same medical condition. The actual distinction in diagnosis (for example, autism versus Asperger's) is less important than recognizing whether your child has an autism spectrum disorder, as the therapies are very similar.

Children with ASD have difficulties with three types of social behavior (these are often called **domains**), including:

- **Social and emotional interaction,** which affects the development of relationships and interactions with family and friends. Common behaviors include solitary play, lack of showing or pointing out objects of interest, and difficulties with non-verbal behaviors. The inability to show affection doesn't mean a child with autism doesn't love or have feelings; she just expresses her emotions in a different way.

- **Restricted interests and repetitive behaviors** that appear to serve no purpose, such as preoccupation with a specific object or abnormal focus on routines or rituals. This may also include body movements such as twirling, arm flapping, rocking, and walking on tiptoes.
- **Communication impairments,** both verbal and non-verbal. Language may be delayed, or language skills may initially develop and then regress. Children with speech issues may repeat words over and over or be unable to initiate or sustain a conversation. Problems with non-verbal communication include lack of pointing or gesturing to objects, inappropriate facial gestures, and the inability to look someone in the eye.

Approximately 1 percent of children have a disorder in the autism spectrum. There is a wide range in degree of impairment. Many of these children have normal intelligence, and others do not. The risk of developing ASD is higher among boys and among children born prematurely. Prematurity itself does not cause autism or the other disorders in the spectrum; it's the complications of prematurity that affect the developing brain that are the cause. Medical conditions that increase the risk of ASD may exist before delivery, such as pre-eclampsia and IUGR (intrauterine growth restriction), or develop after birth, such as intraventricular hemorrhage (IVH) and infection. Premature babies who don't experience any of these complications are not at increased risk for autism.

Genetics also play a role, but you should not blame yourself if your child develops an autism spectrum disorder. Genetics influence everything—birth weight, how your baby responds to medications, and even if she develops bronchopulmonary dysplasia. It's no one's fault—we all pass 50 percent of our genetic material on to our children and hope for the best.

Vaccines most definitely do not cause autism. Many studies have shown there is no association between the two.

To have ASD, a child must have problems in all three social domains. Because language and social skills are developing in the first few years, the diagnosis is typically made only after 18 months adjusted age, although some experts are studying whether autism spectrum disorders can be diagnosed earlier. Screening questionnaires are available. (See www.preemieprimer.com.) Behaviors that are the most concerning include the following:

- **Lack of interest in other children.**
- **Never using an index finger to point out objects or indicate interest in something.**
- **Not bringing objects to a parent.**
- **Not imitating behaviors, such as a funny face.**
- **Not responding to her name.**
- **Not looking at objects pointed out by a parent.**

Your baby's primary care provider should screen your baby for autism at 18 months and again at 24 months (adjusted age). If there's any concern, referral to a specialist, generally a developmental pediatrician or a pediatric neurologist, will be recommended.

Many premature babies exhibit some behaviors that are seen with autism spectrum disorder, such as arm flapping or fear of loud noises. These symptoms are also seen with other conditions. For example, abnormal movements and postures may be caused by cerebral palsy or an isolated motor delay, and fear of loud noises may represent a sensory processing disorder. The key distinguishing factor between other conditions and the autism spectrum is social interaction. A baby who can smile at a socially appropriate time, point at what she likes or wants, and shows interest in what's going on in her environment is unlikely to have autism.

The following blood tests may be performed to rule out other conditions that can have symptoms similar to autism:

- Lead levels
- Thyroid function
- Certain genetic conditions

The most successful approach for a child with an autism spectrum disorder involves educational programming and working with an experienced occupational and speech therapist to learn new behaviors to improve function. Playgroups that model typical social behavior may be beneficial. Some families also find that animal therapy, specifically interacting with dogs or horses, is helpful. Many of the therapies for sensory processing disorder are also used as therapy for autistic conditions.

Many university hospitals and large medical groups have specific autism programs involving multiple specialists. Even if you can't attend one of these programs on a regular basis, an initial consultation and periodic evaluations can be helpful. These doctors, nurses, and therapists

Our society thrives on an artificial idea of perfection—being the best is presented as the only option. Many parents are competitive and delight in stories that extol superlative attributes such as the earliest walker, best eater, or longest naps. As their children get older, the parents brag about grades (those annoying honor roll bumper stickers), athletic prowess, or musical ability. I remember hearing a friend talking about Yale (her child was six), and all I could think was, "I hope Oliver and Victor learn to eat one day."

What I do know is that all premature babies are amazing. They try so hard, struggling to do what we take for granted: breathing, eating, and staying warm. They give it their all, not only in the hospital but for years to come, and they triumph under the most difficult circumstances. I look at our children and I think of how hard they worked to get off the ventilator or how they struggled to crawl. If I looked at them in another way I would see a tremor, asthma, and cerebral palsy, but instead I see smiles, somersaults, and wonderful personalities. I guess it's all perspective.

When drawn into the competition of modern-day parenting, I often remind myself of a Bob Dylan quote, "A man is a success if he gets up in the morning and goes to bed at night and in between he does what he wants." That's the life I want for my boys.

are aware of the latest research and the best therapists, and they can help you identify federal, state, and community resources.

Be wary of any practitioner who promises a cure and of anyone who's trying to sell you a product. It's hard to be an unbiased physician or therapist *and* a salesperson at the same time. Nutrition-based therapies, detoxification, and intravenous therapies have not proven to be effective and in many cases can be harmful. It's not wrong to hold out hope for improvement—with the right therapies, many children make incredible progress. However, developmental disorders like autism cannot be cured. In reality, medicine cures relatively few conditions (think of asthma or diabetes), but most medical conditions can typically be managed very effectively.

26

Preemies Get Diaper Rash, Too

Friends and other parents are more than happy to give their well-meaning advice about baby care; however, many premature babies have unique needs.

Skin Care

Your premature baby has very sensitive skin, so it's best to limit contact with chemicals including lotions and bath products. A few skin care basics for premature babies:

- **Water is often enough to clean.** Soap is for dirt, and your baby is unlikely to be playing in the sand or the mud until she is at least a year old. These early baths are more about relaxing and getting used to the water than they are about actual cleaning. If needed, use a mild, fragrance-free glycerin soap, like Neutrogena, and a mild baby shampoo.
- **Your baby doesn't need a bath every day.** If it's fun for both of you then go ahead, but some babies with sensory issues dislike being wet. (See chapter 25.) If bathing is uncomfortable, discuss how you should proceed with your baby's primary care provider and an occupational therapist.

- **Don't use any powders,** including talcum powder or cornstarch, unless specifically prescribed by your baby's primary care provider. Powders form a dust cloud your baby can inhale.

- **Don't use any products with fragrance,** including laundry detergent. Fragrance, whether it's a plant extract or not, is a chemical and a potential source of irritation. Unscented products contain fewer chemicals. Specific baby detergents are usually not needed.

- **Use an extra rinse cycle** to get all the detergent out of clothes, sheets, and towels if your baby seems sensitive.

- **Throw away fabric softener and dryer sheets.** These products leave a lot of chemical residue. You will save money—and remember, the hospital didn't use fabric softener, so why start now?

- **Natural doesn't mean safe.** For example, ingredients such as lavender and tea tree oil are found in many baby products, but they can be irritating to delicate skin and trigger allergic reactions.

From his first bath in the NICU at 34 weeks, it was clear that Victor had a problem with being wet. I thought maybe it was the hospital, but at home he screamed, arched his back, and stiffened up every time he got wet. Interestingly, I could hold him over the sink and wash his hair, but if a drop of water went below his ears he panicked.

I asked his pediatrician. The answer, "He is five months old, he doesn't *need* a bath."

Of course he didn't need a bath. He was an infant and on oxygen, he wasn't playing outside in the mud! Why stress his nervous system with an unpleasant sensation that isn't even necessary? Out went the bath.

However, since he had bad cradle cap I would wrap him tightly in a towel, burrito-style (as they had in the NICU), and wash his hair carefully over the bathroom sink. This wrapping kept his hands to his midline, helped keep him organized neurologically, and also kept his body dry. I sang (because he seemed to like that the most) and fussed over him as if he were at a spa.

Twice a week we did our spa ritual, and each time I gradually moved the cloth a millimeter down his neck. It took over a year, but by 18 months he was sitting and playing in the tub as if he were born to swim. Now I can't get him out of the bathtub!

If your baby is on oxygen, pay particular attention to the skin under the adhesives on her cheeks. It can become irritated and is more susceptible to breakdown. Make each adhesive patch last as long as possible— until they're practically falling off the skin, if you can. If you need to remove a patch and it doesn't peel away easily, soak it with a wet facecloth with a small amount of baby shampoo to weaken the adhesive.

Cradle Cap

Cradle cap (also called **seborrheic dermatitis**) is a condition in which thick, crusty, greasy, yellow scales grow on your baby's head. Sometimes it can extend down to the ears and the eyebrows. While the exact cause is unknown, one popular medical theory is exposure to the mother's hormones during pregnancy, which can trigger an excess production of oil.

Cradle cap does not look nice, but it doesn't itch and is harmless. It probably bothers you more than it bothers your baby. It will eventually clear up on its own, but you can also wash your baby's hair with a mild baby shampoo and loosen the scales with a soft toothbrush before rinsing. Do not pick at the scales. To further soften the scales, some people recommend rubbing a few drops of baby oil, mineral oil, or olive oil into the scalp before shampooing, making their removal easier. Special cradle cap shampoos are available, and some babies respond better to these products than to regular baby shampoo.

If cradle cap persists more than a few months or gets inflamed, bleeds, or spreads beyond the scalp, you should have your baby evaluated by her primary care provider (PCP), because there are other skin conditions that can look like cradle cap.

When cradle cap persists for more than a year or two, it's probably dandruff. They look similar, although dandruff is partly due to a mild yeast infection in the scalp and is frequently itchy. Medicated shampoos like Head and Shoulders can be very effective, but sometimes a prescription product is needed. Never use a medicated shampoo unless specifically recommended by your baby's PCP.

Diaper Rash

When the diaper area is red and inflamed, it's called diaper rash. There are two causes:

- **Irritation from urine and stool touching the skin.** The rash is pink or red (like a sunburn) and only appears where the skin touches the diaper (so the creases are unaffected).
- **A yeast infection.** The skin is a much brighter or even a dusky red, the rash involves the skin creases, and there may be smaller islands of rash on the uninvolved skin.

Any situation that encourages excess moisture in the diaper area can lead to either kind of diaper rash. Common contributing factors are friction, leaving a wet diaper on for too long, and using plastic overpants on top of the diapers. Yeast infections develop when the bacteria in the bowel changes, which allows yeast to overgrow. Antibiotics (taken by the baby or a breast-feeding mom) can alter the bacteria in the bowel. Breast-feeding, which promotes healthy bowel bacteria, is protective against yeast infections. The best preventive measure against diaper rash is keeping your baby's bottom as dry as possible.

Gentle cleaning after every bowel movement is important, but it's not necessary to wipe after simply urinating. When your baby has a diaper rash, use a wet facecloth, because diaper wipes are irritating on raw skin. Let your baby go diaper free as much as possible, as the circulating air is very helpful. A barrier ointment should be used to protect her skin from further irritation while it heals. Vaseline and A&D, common diaper rash ointments, contain petrolatum, which is a petroleum derivative and potentially flammable. They should not be used if your baby is on oxygen. In addition, many parents don't want to put a petroleum product on their baby's skin, so a petrolatum-free zinc oxide ointment or lanolin, a thick paste-like ointment derived from the grease on wool, are options.

When using an ointment for diaper rash, apply it generously to form a physical barrier. Don't try to remove the ointment each time you change the diaper; rather, dab your baby's bottom with a wet cloth to clean any urine or stool and then reapply. If your baby is very soiled, you may have to soak her in a tub. You can soak your baby frequently if it's comforting. Adding some oatmeal to the water may be soothing. (You can use a commercially prepared oatmeal bath product or make it yourself by grinding one cup of regular oatmeal in a food processor or blender, putting it in a nylon stocking knotted at the top, and placing it in her bathwater.)

Contact your baby's PCP if you suspect a yeast infection, if there are open sores, or if there is no improvement within 48 hours.

Eczema

Eczema is an itchy, red rash. It may form blisters, and the skin can break open and scab. The skin may also appear dry. Eczema is most commonly due to skin irritation or an allergic reaction to chemicals, such as soap or laundry detergent; however, for 20 percent of children, eczema may be the result of a food allergy.

If your baby has eczema, make sure you're not using any products with fragrance or that contain tea tree oil. Consider switching to a mild detergent, such as Dreft, for your baby's clothes, sheets, and towels, and run everything through an extra rinse cycle. Stop all skin care products including soaps and shampoos. Lanolin can trigger allergic reactions, although this is very rare.

In addition to removing the trigger and using good skin care, keep your baby's fingernails short to limit irritation when she scratches. Apply a moisturizing cream such as Lubriderm, Eucerin, or Cetaphil (Lubriderm Daily Moisture–Fragrance Free and Cetaphil Moisturizing Lotion are petrolatum free). For best results, apply right after a bath to help trap in moisture. If you want a natural alternative, you can use a small amount of olive oil. Apply the cream or oil anytime throughout the day if your baby's skin appears raw or irritated.

Contact your baby's PCP if her skin is not improving with these conservative measures or if she's having trouble sleeping, the rash bleeds, or looks like it could be getting infected (yellow drainage or honey-colored crusts). Treatments may include a steroid ointment (reduces the itch and treats the allergy component) and an antihistamine (medication that helps control itching). Antibiotics may be needed if the skin is infected.

If meticulous skin care and prescribed treatments are not helping, a food allergy may be the cause. (See chapter 24.) Your PCP may recommend allergy testing. Changing your baby's diet should help, and you should see improvement within two weeks of dietary modifications. Discuss any changes you plan to make in your baby's diet with her PCP. Typical dietary changes include:

- **Eliminating eggs, nuts, milk, and shellfish from your diet if breast-feeding.**
- **Switching from a regular milk-based formula to a hydrolyzed formula if your baby is formula-fed.** (See chapter 24.) Don't use soy formula as it can also trigger food allergies.
- **Eliminating eggs, nuts, milk, and shellfish from your child's diet.** Talk with her PCP about other sources of calcium and nutrients and how and when to reintroduce these foods.

Some babies and children with food allergies will also need prescription medications (steroids and antihistamines) to help control symptoms.

Sun Protection

Exposure to the sun can cause painful burns and skin cancer. The best protection is covering your baby with loose-fitting tight-weave clothing and a wide-brim hat. Many strollers also have effective sunshades. The sun is most powerful between 10 AM and 4 PM, so it's very important to be most vigilant during that time. If your baby is on oxygen, you also want to avoid being in direct sunlight for long periods of time as this can raise the temperature in the oxygen tank, which is potentially hazardous.

If your baby is six months adjusted age or older, exposed skin should be covered liberally with a broad-spectrum sunscreen—an SPF 15 or greater (the label should say UVA and UVB protection) or a complete sunblock (such as zinc oxide or titanium dioxide). A small amount of sunscreen on exposed hands and feet is acceptable for babies less than six months old. The best choice if you're concerned about chemicals is zinc oxide or titanium dioxide. These products work by physically covering the skin (like clothes) and are not absorbed.

Don't use aerosol sunscreens because your baby can inhale the mist. Aerosols should never be used around oxygen, as the propellant is flammable.

Insect Repellant

Not only are bug bites itchy, but mosquitoes can transmit West Nile virus and deer ticks can transmit Lyme disease. If your baby is two months old (adjusted age) or younger, insect repellants are not recommended, so the only option is to stay indoors or use mosquito netting. Insect repellants should be considered if your baby is older than two months and at risk for bites. Choose a pump product, dispense the repellant into your hand, and then apply to your child. Avoid areas around the eyes and mouth, also the hands in babies and younger children who may put their hands in their mouths. Don't use aerosol sprays, and keep your baby away from burning mosquito coils, as the fumes can irritate the lungs. Wristbands with insect repellants are ineffective, so don't waste your money.

There are two choices for insect repellant:

- **DEET-containing repellants,** which are effective against mosquitoes and ticks. Don't use a product with more than 30 percent DEET (N,N-diethyl-3-methylbenzamide). Concentrations around 10 percent are effective for approximately two hours and a 24 percent concentration provides an average of four and a half hours of protection. DEET-containing products should only be applied once a day. Do not use products that combine DEET and sunscreen, as sunscreen needs to be applied repeatedly. DEET is not water soluble, so unlike sunscreen it doesn't need to be reapplied after swimming.

- **DEET-free insect repellants.** Only products with eucalyptus oil (such as Repel) are effective against both mosquitoes and ticks. Eucalyptus oil repellants work for about two hours; however, they're *not recommended* for children three years and younger. Other effective DEET-free products contain 2 percent soybean oil or picaridin, but they're only effective against mosquitoes. Soybean oil–containing repellants can be used when your baby is two months adjusted age or older. Other DEET-free alternatives, such as lavender oil or products with citronella or peppermint oil, are not recommended because they only provide protection from mosquitoes for 30 minutes or less. Exercise the same caution applying DEET-free products to areas around the eyes and mouth and the hands.

Sleep Habits

The first step is deciding where your baby will sleep. Studies suggest that sudden infant death syndrome (SIDS) is lower when your newborn sleeps in the same room with you. When you feel comfortable moving your baby to a nursery will depend on her medical concerns as well as your personal beliefs. However, if your baby is on an apnea monitor or pulse oximeter, she must be close enough so you can hear and respond quickly to an alarm. A baby monitor is a good idea no matter where your baby sleeps so you can keep track of her as you move around your house. Many parents prefer a video monitor, especially if their baby is on oxygen. If your baby is on an apnea monitor, make sure there is no electrical interference from your baby monitor.

To reduce the risk of sudden infant death syndrome (SIDS), all babies should sleep on their backs on a firm mattress with tight-fitting sheets. Don't use bumpers or pillows. A fitted sleeper outfit is best for warmth, but if a blanket is needed, it should be firmly tucked in over the lower half of your baby at the foot of the crib or bassinet. The American Academy of Pediatrics advises against co-sleeping due to the potential risks of in-

When Oliver was starting to roll over and Victor's reflux had improved enough that we could lay him down with the mattress elevated, we transitioned the boys to cribs in our bedroom. It was a very tight fit, but we managed. The only problem—Oliver would only sleep in the crib with the side railing pulled *halfway* up. When he started sitting up we knew we had to raise the railing all the way, but he screamed until he threw up and then would cry again, often dropping his oxygen levels. His screaming upset Victor (even if he were in a different room) so much that Victor would cry and start to vomit. If we waited until Oliver was asleep to put him in the crib, somehow he would sense the transfer and commence the cycle of crying and vomiting. We read countless books on the subject, and many well-meaning parents told us about their surefire ways of getting their children to sleep in a crib. We tried several, always with the same result.

So after trying our best, we gave up. We sold their cribs and bought a firm queen-size mattress for the floor of the nursery (which up until now had served only as a diaper-changing/oxygen storage area). Even then, when we tried to leave the room the cycle of crying and vomiting would start. By this time, Oliver had been hospitalized twice with pneumonia, and these admissions clearly affected his ability to be in any room without a parent. Though co-sleeping is not recommended by the American Academy of Pediatrics, we didn't seem to have any other option. Oliver could pull himself up to sit, so he could not be in a crib with the railing halfway up, and under no circumstances could we leave the room with him in a bed. So for the next year and a half we all slept on the mattress on the floor. By now they were both off of their monitors, and the mattress was in the middle of the room, with no headboard and tight-fitting sheets. Sometimes you just have to do the best with what you have.

fant death. Pillows, extra sheets, and comforters all pose a suffocation risk, and a baby can also get stuck in the headboard slats, between the mattress and the headboard, or between the mattress and the wall. In addition, if your baby is on an apnea monitor, your breathing may confuse the monitor.

Options for sleeping in your room are a bassinet next to your bed or a co-sleeper, which is a bassinet that attaches to your bed but is open on your side so you can easily see and touch your baby. You can also set up her crib in your room. If you decide to get a bassinet or co-sleeper, choose one that is rated to at least 15 pounds so you can use it for many months. Once your baby is too heavy for the bassinet/co-sleeper or can roll over, she'll need to sleep in a crib.

Getting your premature baby to develop good sleep habits can be challenging. She may need more frequent feedings and not give clear cues that she's tired. Because she may be used to the noise of the NICU, you may find that your baby sleeps better with soft background noise (classical music or white noise, like the sound of rain). Once your baby gets older, she may fuss and cry when left in her bassinet or crib. Many experts advocate rubbing her back and trying to soothe her without picking her up. Talk with your baby's PCP about the best approach for your baby, as you must also consider her medical conditions. For example, if your baby is on oxygen, leaving her alone to fuss or cry may not be an option.

Plagiocephaly

Plagiocephaly is a condition in which a baby's skull develops a flat spot on the side or the back of the head. It's increasing in prevalence as babies now sleep on their backs at all times to reduce the risk of SIDS. A premature baby has a softer skull at birth, so she's at greater risk. In addition, many premature babies have motor delays and take longer to learn to roll over, so they spend more time on their backs. Torticollis, an abnormal tightening of the neck muscles on one side, also plays a role, as the head is continually in one position. For some babies, torticollis may be related to reflux, as facing in one direction may help them cope with the discomfort. However, prolonged time in this position can stiffen the muscles involved. Torticollis may also be a sign of cerebral palsy.

Plagiocephaly can often be prevented by letting your baby spend time on her tummy every day while she's awake (as long as you're watching) and limiting the amount of time she spends in her car seat, because this position also places pressure on the back of the head. Periodically alternate the way her head faces when she's sleeping on her back. If she

Within a few months of coming home, it became apparent that Victor always had his head turned toward his right shoulder. At first I thought it was a preference, but I soon realized his head was developing a pronounced oblique shape and, because his neck muscles were so tight on one side, it was physically difficult for him to turn his head in the other direction. He had torticollis. We had done plenty of tummy time, but as he could not lift his head very well he often just lay there with his head turned to his right.

I started placing a roll under his right shoulder, taping it to his clothes so that every time I laid him down or placed him in a swing his head could only roll to the left, stretching the abnormally taut muscles on his right. Every time I picked him up I turned his head to his left, and in any downtime I massaged his tightened and twisted right side, hoping to relax the muscles even a little. Once he started getting some head control, I would place him in a baby chair in front of the TV, but angled in such a way that he could only see the screen if he used his weaker muscles and turned his head to his left side. We did this for 15 minutes three times a day. Gradually his left side strengthened and his head evened out. It's still shaped a little oddly at the back, but he has so much hair it's impossible to tell just by looking at it. His right side is still tight, but he has developed so much control over his muscles that he manages just fine, although he still loves to have his neck massaged. The biggest negative remnant seems to be a TV addiction, which I hear is also a problem for many other parents who never experienced torticollis.

seems to always keep her head in one direction, she may have torticollis, so she should be checked by her PCP.

While plagiocephaly can often be corrected by paying close attention to head position, some babies will need intervention. This may include a band or helmet that serves as a mold, encouraging the head to grow symmetrically. If torticollis is present, the cause must be identified and the stiffness treated, typically with physical therapy and stretching exercises.

PART SIX

Other Things You Should Know

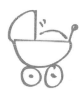

27

What No One Else Will Tell You

Is My Baby in the Right Hospital?

There are some hospital-related factors that make a difference in outcome for premature babies, including:

- **Having your baby born where she will be getting her care.** Premature babies transferred after birth face more challenges than babies born down the hall from the intensive care unit. If there's a known chance you could deliver prematurely, it's best to be in a medical center with an intensive care unit that can meet your baby's needs.
- **A nursery that cares for 100 or more babies a year.** Looking after premature babies requires specialized training *and* experience.
- **A neonatal intensive care unit where the health care professionals are NIDCAP certified.** NIDCAP stands for Newborn Individualized Developmental Care and Assessment Program, and staff who have graduated from these programs are taught to handle premature babies in a way that lessens the impact on the nervous system.

Preventing Medical Errors

An unfortunate part of medical care is medical errors, and the most common errors involve medications. To reduce these errors, be aware of the five "rights" of medication safety. When administering medication, a nurse or parent should check for:

- **The right medication.** Know every medication, the side effects, and why it's needed. In the hospital, IV bags and syringes should be labeled to avoid mix-ups—one syringe filled with a clear liquid looks just like another. Ask to be informed every time a new medication is started, keep a list, and maintain the same vigilance at home.
- **The right dose.** Due to a premature baby's small size, many medications require very specific calculations to achieve the correct dose. Doses also need to be adjusted frequently (increasing the risk for error) due to weight gain. Premature babies are also less tolerant of dosing errors.
- **The right time.** Ask how many times a day a medication is given.
- **The right route.** By mouth or intravenous (IV), injection in the muscle (intramuscular, or IM) or the skin (subcutaneous, or SC).
- **The right patient.** This is self-explanatory, but parents with multiples need to be especially vigilant.

Try to understand how each medication fits into your baby's health care and what doctors are looking for to prove the medication is actually working. Doctors and nurses are a great source of this information, but many hospitals have a dedicated pediatric pharmacist who can provide a wealth of information.

If your baby is in a teaching hospital, be especially vigilant from the end of June through the end of August. This is when new interns and residents start. Studies show that inexperience factors into medication and other medical errors.

It is important to be as careful at home as at the hospital. Some tips to reduce medication errors at home:

- **Double check every prescription at the pharmacy,** as 12 percent of prescriptions written by hand and 6 percent of electronic prescriptions contain errors.
- **Prepare and administer at least one dose of each medication prior to discharge** (for medications started during a hospital admission).
- **Ask for written information about each medication, including dose, how often it's to be taken, and side effects.** Many of the instructions are difficult to remember and easily misunderstood.
- **Ask about potential side effects, risks, and interactions with other medications.**
- **Ask how the medications should be given in relationship with meals,** for example, on an empty stomach, with water, or with food.
- **Ask what to do if you miss a dose.** No one thinks they will forget, but it happens. Some medications should be given as soon as the error is realized, but with others the missed dose should be skipped altogether.
- **Double check the label before giving each dose at home.** Keep your baby's medication separate from other prescriptions and over-the-counter medications to avoid mix-ups, especially for doses given late at night.
- **Bring all the current medications to every follow-up visit,** so your doctor knows exactly what your baby is taking. A list might be easier, but many drug names are very similar and it's possible to make an error transcribing the name or dose.

Conflict

There may be times when you disagree with your baby's providers, feel an issue is not being addressed, or are unhappy with the medical care.

After five years of daily medications for low thyroid and asthma as well as a revolving door of antibiotics, antivirals, and reflux medications, I felt I had it all under control. I had a routine, a spot in a kitchen cupboard for pills and inhalers, special syringes to measure liquids, labeled pill cutters for each medication, and a mortar and pestle. There were no missed doses and no surprises. But as with any situation that seems to be running without a hitch, I was vulnerable to the creep of complacency.

My husband received a new prescription for a heart medication. For a while it stayed in his medicine cabinet, but somehow it migrated to the little cupboard with the boys' medications. First it was a shelf above. "That's okay," I said. "I'm a doctor, really, what kind of mistake am I going to make?" Eventually, the medication found its way to the lower shelf.

One night I grabbed Victor's thyroid medication, just as always, opened the bottle, and handed him his medication, a white pill. As he reached for it, I saw out of the corner of my eye that the shape was wrong. I was holding one of Tony's pills.

The surge of panic left me physically ill. What if I had given him that pill? I knew the consequences of giving an adult-strength heart medication to a five-year-old boy. Shaking, I grabbed Tony's medication, walked to our bathroom, and placed it on the highest self. We talked about keeping one cabinet for Victor and one for Oliver and checking for errant bottles every time we opened the door. I insisted the boys learn the label of every new medication. They can't read all the words, but they know their own names. We look at the bottle together, re-read the label, and make sure we are following the instructions correctly. Right medication, right time, right dose, right route, right patient. Every time. It takes about one minute.

Conflict usually arises from a combination of communication difficulties and fear.

While your concerns are valid, it's important to remember that conflict is never productive. Although there may be times you can change the situation, most often the best option (and possibly the only one) is to find a resolution. Escalating the situation is never productive, but neither is silently giving in. You may have a good reason to be upset, but you may also have misinterpreted what was said, and you will not know this if you don't communicate.

Conflict may result from:

- **Personality-based issues.** Some health care professionals will mesh better with your personal style than others. If you're having difficulty interacting with a specific provider, speak with one of the neonatologists or pediatricians, the charge nurse, or the social worker. You are not the first parent to have ever experienced conflict in a hospital, so they will almost always have productive suggestions. If the conflict arises in a doctor's office, discuss your concerns with the clinic manager and the doctor. Some parents can also switch providers, but that's not always an option, depending on where you live. If you're having interaction problems with a specialist, discuss the issues with your baby's primary care provider. They are also your advocate.

- **Disagreement over medical care or feeling that the staff is not doing everything possible.** Many times this conflict stems from a communication problem. Complex information and the stress of the situation can make it almost impossible to absorb all that is happening. Be upfront about your concerns and make sure you understand the medical plan to your satisfaction. In the NICU, ask for regular team meetings so you can stay apprised of your baby's condition. It's important to advocate for your baby, but you also have to remember that the medical team has a lot of experience and is trying to do the best thing for your baby. The doctors, nurses, and therapists who are caring for your baby are making their recommendations in good faith. It takes devoted staff to work in a neonatal intensive care unit and generally these are some of the best nurses and doctors in the facility. Keep in mind that many problems don't have an easy solution.

If you're not satisfied after a team meeting, you can ask for another opinion, both in the hospital or as an out-patient from a different specialist. A good place to look for a second opinion is from a doctor on staff at a large university medical center. In the hospital you can also involve a patient advocate.

Doctors, nurses, and therapists should be able to explain why a particular therapy is or is not necessary. It's important to speak up when you're concerned, but you should also seriously consider why you disagree. Do your own research, but be wary of information from anyone who guarantees success, has not published their results in a respected medical journal, or states that they are the only person in the country who can do a procedure.

Putting Tests into Perspective

Tests, such as blood work, X-rays, and scans, can be helpful in making a diagnosis and monitoring therapy. While it's easy for us to have blood taken or hold still for an X-ray, this is not the case for a baby. Tests also have consequences. Not only do blood tests contribute to anemia, but it's frightening to be held down, and the needle hurts. X-rays and CT scans are associated with radiation, and some tests require sedation because holding very still is essential for accurate results.

The most important question to ask is, "How will this test change my baby's care?" If the treatment will be the same regardless of the results, perhaps the test can be avoided. The second question is, "What are the risks of the test?" The potential benefits must clearly outweigh the risks.

The Missed Pregnancy Experience

When you deliver prematurely, you may miss out on a lot of the fun part of pregnancy and having a newborn. You may deliver long before your baby shower is even organized or be too sick or stressed to participate with friends and family to have a baby shower while you're hospitalized. If your baby is in the NICU, the idea of a shower or a celebration may simply not occur to your friends. Also, you may not feel like being around a lot of people and answering emotionally difficult questions.

Sometimes family members and friends hold back on sending gifts, afraid to give something in case the outcome is bad. However, they don't understand that if things go terribly wrong after delivery, some extra sleepers and a receiving blanket are inconsequential.

Your baby should be unconditionally celebrated. While you may not feel like a shower or a party, a gift to welcome your baby is appropriate. Register, if you were planning on doing that before you knew you would deliver prematurely. If friends and family ask what to get you, here are a few things you might say:

- "Whatever you were planning on getting me before you knew I would deliver prematurely."
- "A food basket, groceries, or meals to freeze." When your baby is in the hospital, there's little time to shop or cook, and eating out, even at hospital cafeterias, gets expensive. Nutritious food is especially important for breast-feeding moms.
- "A stuffed animal would be very dear to us. We can place it in the incubator (or crib) or have it waiting at home."
- "A great diaper bag."
- "Preemie clothes." It can be comforting to take the clothes home and wash them.
- "A baby journal or scrapbook."
- "Get vaccinated or give blood in honor of my baby."

Getting the Most Out of Your Doctor's Appointment

Your baby will have a lot of appointments in her first few years. There are many ways to make these visits easier on both you and your baby:

- **Always ask for the first appointment of the day.** Everyone is fresh and ready to go. In addition, sick children tend to be worked in later in the day, so in the early morning you're less likely to expose your child to a waiting room full of sick children. If the first appointment is not available, get a morning appointment or the first appointment in the afternoon.
- **Arrive at least 15 minutes early for every appointment** to check in and complete the paperwork.

When Victor had his tonsils removed, I was given a handout the day of discharge. I'm sure the nurse told me it was important follow-up information, and I'm sure I rolled my eyes. After all, I'm a surgeon—what's a handout going to tell me about a little old tonsillectomy?

The first few days of recovery were rough, but Victor got better each day. However, on the seventh day he took a turn for the worse. He had a fever, couldn't swallow, and had a foul smell from his mouth. Maybe he had an infection? Worried, I called the doctor's office and asked to speak with the nurse.

I explained Victor's symptoms, that *I was Dr. Gunter*, and that I was sure he had an infection. "Should we go to the emergency room or can you fit us into a clinic appointment?" I asked.

"Did you read the handout you were given on discharge?" she asked.

"Well, of course I did," I lied.

"Then you know fever, sore throat, and a foul smell are classic signs that the scab in his throat is coming off, which happens on day seven." She paused for effect.

Mortified, I managed to mumble, "Just checking," before hanging up.

Since then I have read every single handout that has been offered to me.

- **Prepare ahead of time for the ophthalmologist.** Your baby will need eye drops and they take 20 or 30 minutes to work. If your baby's ophthalmologist cares for many premature babies, their office will be busy as there will always be new NICU graduates needing eye exams. You may be in the office for one to two hours, so bring enough food, diapers, wipes, and whatever else you may need.

- **Find out your provider's policy for patients who show up early.** If you're early and the person ahead of you is late, there is a good chance you may be seen sooner. It's a gamble, but you'd be surprised by how many people are late or simply don't show at all.

- **Get to know the office staff.** They control the appointments. Don't try to ingratiate yourself, but treat them with respect. If you're the type of person who gives a gift to your hairdresser at holiday time, think about giving your providers and their staff a small gift as well. Home baking is perfectly acceptable, but even a card with a picture of your baby will do nicely.

- **If you need to cancel an appointment, call 48 hours in advance.**
- **Plan ahead of time for your appointments.** Write down what you want to say and practice at home. If you have a lot to cover, or felt rushed the last time, ask for a longer appointment. Doctors can bill your insurance for their time. This way your baby gets the care she needs, your doctor gets paid, and no one runs late.
- **Read everything you are given.**

Epilogue

~~~~~~

If We Did It,
So Can You

> I worried so much about the future when my boys were in the hospital, and that fear did not dissipate when they came home. Would they sit? Walk? Talk? It was easy to feel hopeless and overwhelmed by the unknown.
>
> However, there was one thing that shone a light in that fog of despair— a poster on the wall in the parents' room. There were 10 or so pictures of NICU graduates, lovely children with beaming smiles. Underneath each picture was a name, gestational age at birth, current age, grade in school, as well as a few lines about their favorite activities. Here on the plain white wall was tangible evidence, heartwarming and hopeful, of life outside an incubator. Living was possible.
>
> I have collected some stories from other premature children as well as Oliver and Victor to serve as my own version of that poster that kept me going.

Katie, age 10. Born at 30 weeks and 6 days weighing 1,723 g (3 lbs, 13 oz).

I was born premature. Because I was an infant, I cannot remember any complications. I'm sure my prematurity caused my parents some grief (especially when I developed an infection in my blood), but there haven't been any long-term effects.

I'm just a normal girl, growing up and learning every day. I am lucky to be an intelligent student with a family who loves me and cares for me.

I like to do many things. I enjoy my dance classes because dance is a good way for me to express myself. I'm in the performing company at my dance studio, so I have the opportunity to participate in performances more often than others. I like to read, and I'm also a good writer and artist. I started knitting a few years ago, and it's something my mom and I like to do together. Recently, I took third place in the Georgia State Spelling Bee. I hope I can be successful when I get older. Being born prematurely was just something that happened to me, and it hasn't changed my life.

Ty, age four. Born at 27 weeks weighing 683 g (1 lb, 8 oz).

I spent six weeks on a ventilator after I was born. My mom and dad were very worried I would never breathe on my own. I spent four months in the NICU and was on oxygen at home for two years. My mom got so tired of lugging my oxygen tank, her purse, and a diaper bag around that she designed her own backpack.

I go to preschool and have been doing speech therapy for three years. Everyone says I am a rambunctious and curious redhead. I am pretty good at cuddling, too.

My lungs don't hold me back anymore. I love to ride my bike, play T-ball, and run around in my Batman cape, pretending I'm a superhero. I love Curious George. My favorite movies are *Monsters vs. Aliens* and *Tinkerbell*. My Dad isn't too thrilled about that last one, but Tink is tiny, stubborn, and fast—just like me! My mom says my stubbornness came in handy in the hospital. I hope she remembers that when I'm in high school!

Julia, age seven. Born at 27 weeks and 5 days weighing 1,076 g (2 lbs, 6 oz).

I was diagnosed with periventricular leukomalacia (PVL) a few weeks after I was born. My mom and dad were very scared and they didn't know what that would mean for me. I have cerebral palsy. While there are some things I have difficulty with, there are a whole bunch of wonderful things I can do.

With the help of my aide and teachers, I am in first grade at school. I love to learn new things. I also love to go on swings, scoot on the floor, walk in my walker, and play with my favorite dolly, Anna. One of my very favorite things is game night with mom and dad. My younger sisters (they are twins, and I sometimes think they were put on this earth just to entertain me) go to bed early on Saturday nights. Because I am the *big* sister, I get to stay up late, sit at the table with my mom and dad, and play one of my favorite games. It's so much fun.

I am a very happy little girl. My mom says I will make the sun shine for you if you are lucky enough to be around me.

Emily and Aaron, twins, age seven. Born at 29 weeks, Emily weighing 1,360 g (2 lbs, 16 oz) and Aaron weighing 1,369 g (3 lbs).

We spent two months in the NICU and our mom says things were pretty scary when we got infected with a virus a few weeks after we were born. It was really hard because it was like starting all over again. The first few years at home we kept our mom and dad on their toes with asthma, reflux, and not wanting to sleep. Just doing our jobs.

Now we are in second grade. We are both doing very well in school. We used to be very afraid of being wet. It took a while to get used to swimming and we took lots of lessons, but now we love the water!

Aaron: I had a lot of fine motor issues that had my teachers and parents concerned in kindergarten, but they've all but disappeared with my hard work. I love to play soccer. I'm not sure what I want to be when I grow up, although I know I don't want to be a doctor, because I don't like to look at blood.

Emily: I'm enjoying my first year of ballet. I love school and everyone comments on how beautifully I print. I would like to be a teacher one day.

Daniel, age seven. Born at 24 weeks weighing 567 g (1 lb, 4 oz).

I spent 20 weeks in the NICU. However, if I had not been born prematurely, my family might never have found me, because I was adopted from the NICU. My mom met me when I was just born and it was love at first sight. I'm lucky to have the most wonderful parents in the whole world.

I spent about 10 weeks on a ventilator and had to have my PDA closed with surgery. My left vocal cord doesn't work very well; my doctors aren't sure if it was from being intubated for so long or from my heart surgery. I have a soft, raspy voice, but it's getting stronger as I grow (like the rest of me). I had laser surgery for my eyes, but I see better with my glasses than my mom does, and she was born at term.

Sometimes I have trouble concentrating and school was getting a bit overwhelming. This year I am repeating first grade. What a difference it has made. I have a lot more confidence and don't mind doing my homework so much anymore.

I recently started Tae Kwon Do. I'm a lot smaller than other boys, so it's nice to do a sport where size doesn't matter. I just earned my white belt, and I'm so happy. (My mom and dad were pretty excited, too.)

I like playing video games, especially Lego Star Wars and Lego Batman. I love to laugh and tell jokes. If something is really funny, I will laugh until I cry.

Aria, age six. Born at 25 weeks and 1 day weighing 567 g (1 lb, 4 oz).

I was on a ventilator after I was born. When I was a month old I caught a viral infection and needed the help of nitric oxide to breathe. That was a very scary time for my mom and dad. I had surgery for my PDA and laser for my eyes. I was also diagnosed with periventricular leukomalacia (PVL). I have cerebral palsy that affects my arms and legs. I use a wheelchair to get around and a G-tube to eat. I have some difficulties seeing because I have cortical visual impairment.

I'm so much more than all of those medical words. I am in kindergarten in a program for children with disabilities. Circle time is my favorite because there is lots of singing and music. I love to listen to Raffi and Laurie Berkner. When I hear a familiar song I have a smile so big it will melt your heart. Sometimes I sing along in my own way. When I hear your voice I will respectfully engage in a conversation with you by looking your way the entire time you speak. I am very polite and well mannered.

I love when my cousins and friends talk and play with me. I also love applause and being outdoors, feeling the wind on my face. I am the biggest daddy's girl and will stop focusing on any and every thing if it means listening to or being with my daddy. I adore him and I think the feeling is mutual.

Oliver, age six. Born at 26 weeks weighing 783 g (1 lb, 11½ oz).

My parents had almost recovered from my rocky start in the NICU when they found out I had a bad heart problem that would require surgery. However, I surprised everyone by being ready to go home after just nine and a half weeks, despite having surgery on my heart valve. I was on oxygen for a year at home. I have been sick many times with pneumonia and also had a second heart surgery. I was admitted to an intensive care unit when I was two and a half with pneumonia and my parents were so worried. My heart and lung problems sometimes make me tired so I like naps. I can usually convince my mom or dad to nap with me on the weekend.

I'm repeating kindergarten this year. My first year in kindergarten was very tiring and I needed to rest. Also, my hands don't always do what I want them to, but having an extra year to practice has helped a lot. I love Pokémon and Bakugan and recently discovered that I love to act. I have been in two plays and I come alive in front of an audience! I want to be an actor and develop the first-ever flying ice-cream truck. I am not going to sell the ice cream, just fly it around.

I'm a very happy boy and people say that my smile is simply indescribable.

Victor, age six. Born at 26 weeks weighing 833 g (1 lb, 13 oz).

I spent 11 weeks in the NICU. I had a lot of problems with reflux. I also have cerebral palsy. I repeated kindergarten this year and it has given me a lot of confidence to make friends, although apparently now I have too many girlfriends. (My dad says I get that from him.)

I'm not supposed to be able to do many of the things that I can do. My doctors are finally beginning to understand that I inherited both of my parent's stubborn genes. My kindergarten teacher said she has never seen a child squeeze out every last drop, like I do. I think that just about sums me up.

It took a lot of practice, but I can jump with two feet and hopscotch like a pro. The monkey bars were very hard for me at first, because my arms don't always do what I want them to, so I often practice until my hands bleed. I have the coolest collection of blisters and calluses, and I'm very proud of them.

I write stories every night and I'm very good at art. I want to be a doctor, an author, an artist, and study killer jellyfish. Only killer jellyfish, not the other kind.

Acknowledgments

I must begin by thanking Dr. Adam Rosenberg from the division of neonatology at University Hospital in Colorado. Without your expert guidance I have no doubt that I would be writing a very different book. I have worked with many doctors over the past 24 years, and you are simply one of the best.

Thank you to all the medical professionals and staff, both in Colorado and in California, who have cared for my boys and me. Special thanks to Dr. Kak-Chen Chan, Dr. Henry Galan, Dr. Jill Davies, Dr. Amnon Goodman, and Dr. Jorge Gutierrez as well as Kami and Stacey, two of the best NICU nurses on the planet.

To Joyce Rosner for her beautiful illustrations and support—not many people are lucky enough to have such a wonderful and talented sister-in-law.

A special thank-you to the families who graciously shared their stories. You and your children are truly inspiring.

To my friends Tania Malik, Maya Creedman, Stephanie Teal, Gail Marks, Jennifer Schmitt, Vilma Velarde, and Cara Willems. You have all carried me in some way or another, and I am so grateful for your love and friendship.

Thank you to Jennifer De La Fuente for your guidance and to Katie McHugh and all the wonderful people at Da Capo.

To my boys for being my reason—words are inadequate to describe my love for you. (Please remember that when you are teenagers.)

And last of all to my husband, Tony. Thank you for standing back until the tornado is over. Well, it's never really over, but sometimes there are breaks in the storm (although you knew that getting into this whole thing).

Contributors

Many thanks to the following experts for their insightful comments and suggestions.

Dr. John Baier MD, FRCPC
Associate Professor of Pediatrics and Child Health
Division of Neonatology
University of Manitoba

Dr. Victor Chernick MD, FRCPC
Professor Emeritus
Department of Pediatrics
University of Manitoba

Dr. Jill Davies MD, FACOG
Associate Professor of Obstetrics and Gynecology
Division of Maternal-Fetal Medicine
University of Colorado Denver School of Medicine

Dr. Eric Eichenwald MD, FAAP
Associate Professor of Pediatrics
Division of Neonatology
Baylor College of Medicine

Dr. Nicole Fallaha MD, FRCSC
Assistant Clinical Professor of Opthalmology
Division of Pediatric Opthalmology
Université de Montréal

Dr. Henry Galan MD, FACOG
Professor of Obstetrics and Gynecology
Division of Maternal-Fetal Medicine
University of Colorado Denver School of Medicine

Dr. Lisa Griffin MD, FAAP
Department of Pediatrics
Division of Pediatric Neurology
Kaiser Permanente, San Francisco

Dr. Dorothea Jenkins MD, FAAP
Associate Professor of Pediatrics
Division of Neonatology
Medical University of South Carolina

Dr. Clark E. Nugent MD, FACOG
Professor of Obstetrics and Gynecology
Division of Maternal-Fetal Medicine
University of Michigan Medical School

Dr. J. Colin Partridge
Professor of Clinical Pediatrics
Division of Neonatology
University of California, San Francisco

Dr. Joseph Polimeni MD, FRCPC
Associate Professor of Psychiatry
University of Manitoba

Dr. Philip E. Putnam MD, FAAP
Professor of Pediatrics
Division of Gastroenterology, Hepatology, and Nutrition
University of Cincinnati

Dr. Adam Rosenberg MD, FAAP
Professor of Pediatrics
Division of Neonatology
University of Colorado Denver School of Medicine

Dr. Jennifer Shine Dyer MD, MPH
Assistant Professor of Pediatrics
Division of Endocrinology
The Ohio State University

Dr. Jennifer Shu MD, FAAP
Pediatrician
Children's Medical Group, P.C.
Co-author, American Academy of Pediatrics publications *Heading Home with Your Newborn, Baby & Child Health*, and *Food Fights*
Atlanta, GA

Tomasz Stasiuk JD
Attorney and Counselor at Law
The Stasiuk Firm, P.C.
Colorado Springs, CO

Appendix

Growth Charts for Boys and Girls

Birth to 36 months: Boys
Length-for-age and Weight-for-age percentiles

NAME _____

RECORD # _____

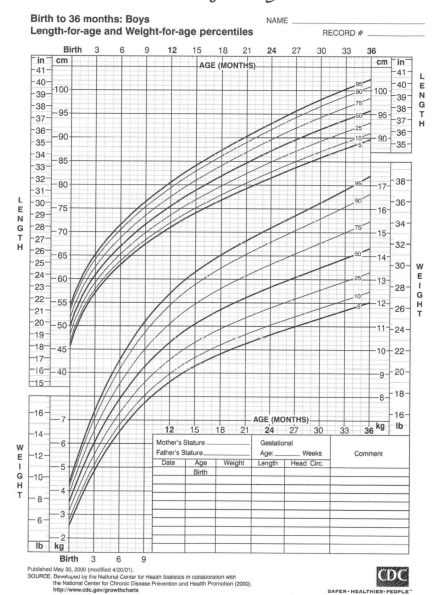

Published May 30, 2000 (modified 4/20/01).
SOURCE: Developed by the National Center for Health Statistics in collaboration with
the National Center for Chronic Disease Prevention and Health Promotion (2000).
http://www.cdc.gov/growthcharts

CDC
SAFER·HEALTHIER·PEOPLE™

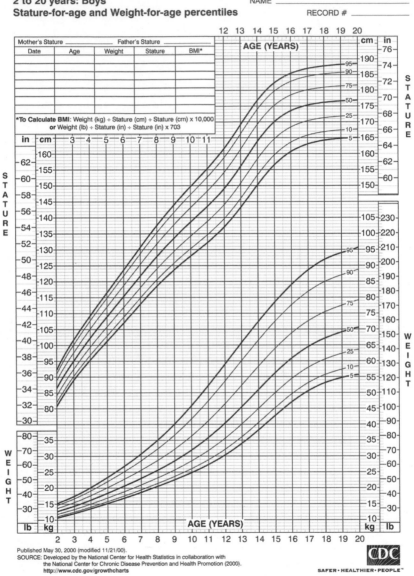

2 to 20 years: Boys
Stature-for-age and Weight-for-age percentiles

NAME _____

RECORD # _____

Published May 30, 2000 (modified 11/21/00).
SOURCE: Developed by the National Center for Health Statistics in collaboration with
the National Center for Chronic Disease Prevention and Health Promotion (2000).
http://www.cdc.gov/growthcharts

SAFER · HEALTHIER · PEOPLE™

Birth to 36 months: Girls
Length-for-age and Weight-for-age percentiles

NAME _____

RECORD # _____

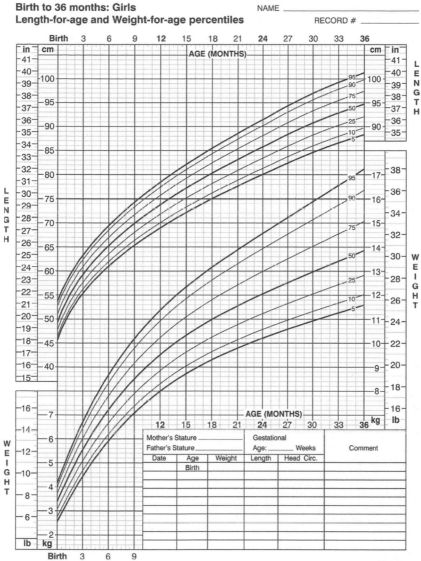

Published May 30, 2000 (modified 4/20/01).
SOURCE: Developed by the National Center for Health Statistics in collaboration with
    the National Center for Chronic Disease Prevention and Health Promotion (2000).
    http://www.cdc.gov/growthcharts

CDC
SAFER · HEALTHIER · PEOPLE™

2 to 20 years: Girls
Stature-for-age and Weight-for-age percentiles

NAME _____

RECORD # _____

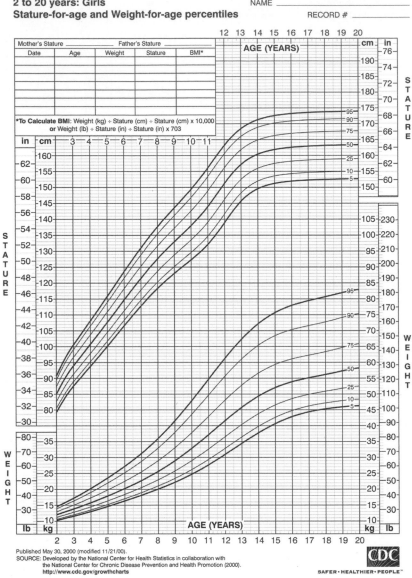

Published May 30, 2000 (modified 11/21/00).
SOURCE: Developed by the National Center for Health Statistics in collaboration with
the National Center for Chronic Disease Prevention and Health Promotion (2000).
http://www.cdc.gov/growthcharts

Glossary

abruption. Bleeding behind the placenta causing premature separation of the placenta, either partially or completely, from the inside of the uterus.

adjusted age. The age of a premature baby adjusted for the degree of prematurity. See also *corrected age*.

alveoli. Tiny air sacs in the lungs where the exchange of oxygen for carbon dioxide occurs.

amniocentesis. A procedure performed during pregnancy in which a needle is inserted through the mother's belly wall into the amniotic sac and a small amount of amniotic fluid is withdrawn for analysis.

amniotic fluid. The fluid that surrounds a baby during pregnancy.

amnion. The innermost membrane of the amniotic sac.

anesthesia. Medication to prevent pain. General anesthesia, often called going to sleep, is unconsciousness resulting from anesthetic drugs that are injected or inhaled.

apnea. Absence of breathing for more than 20 seconds or a shorter pause in breathing that is associated with a drop in blood oxygen level or heart rate.

arrhythmia. Irregular heartbeat.

autonomic nervous system. The part of the nervous system that controls bodily functions not under conscious control, such as heart rate, blood pressure, and sweating.

back transport. Transfer of a premature baby from a level III NICU to a level II nursery closer to home.

barium swallow. A test involving drinking a liquid called barium that can be detected by X-rays. A barium swallow provides information about the anatomy of the esophagus and stomach.

bilirubin. A yellow substance in the blood produced when old red blood cells are recycled. Bilirubin is a toxin and is removed from the blood by the liver and gallbladder.

bili blanket. A blanket with special lights that deliver phototherapy to treat elevated bilirubin levels. Though BiliBlanket is a product name specific to the General Electric brand, the term *bili blanket* is often used for any similar device.

bili lights. Overhead lamps that emit the specific wavelength of light effective for phototherapy treatment of elevated bilirubin levels.

bronchi. Larger airways in the lungs.

bronchioles. Smaller airway in the lungs. They connect the bronchi with the alveoli.

bronchopulmonary dysplasia (BPD). A chronic lung disease caused by prematurity. BPD is characterized by fewer alveoli with thicker walls and inflammation.

cardiopulmonary resuscitation (CPR). A combination of mouth-to-mouth resuscitation (rescue breathing) and chest compressions for the emergency treatment of cardiac arrest. CPR does not restart the heart, but rather keeps blood flowing to the heart and the brain until medical interventions can be mobilized to try to restart the heart.

cerclage. A stitch to strengthen the cervix.

cervix. The lower portion of the uterus, connected to the vagina. The cervix dilates during labor to allow delivery of the baby from the uterus.

central line. An intravenous placed in a large vein in the arm, neck, chest, or groin. These large veins are closer to the heart than the smaller veins in the hands, feet, and scalp.

central nutrition. A method of delivering all the body's nutritional needs via a central line.

cerebellum. The lowermost portion of the brain. It is involved in coordinating movement, balance, and muscle tone.

cerebral cortex. The outermost layer of the brain. It controls the brains higher functions including thought, memory, emotion, movement, speech, and vision. The cerebral cortex is folded into bulges and grooves visible on the surface of the cerebrum and cerebellum.

cerebrospinal fluid (CSF). The fluid that bathes and nourishes the brain and spinal cord.

cerebrum. The largest part of the brain. The cerebrum controls thinking, emotion, sight, speech, hearing, smell, touch, and voluntary movement. It is divided into two halves called hemispheres.

cervical insufficiency. A cervix that measures 2.5 cm or less in length by ultrasound in the second trimester of pregnancy.

chorioamnionitis. Infection of the membranes, placenta, and amniotic fluid.

chorion. The outermost membrane of the amniotic sac.

chronological age. The age of a premature baby calculated from the day of birth.

CMV (cytomegalovirus). A common virus that causes minor symptoms for most adults and children but can seriously affect a developing baby in the womb. A premature baby may develop a much more serious illness if infected.

colostrum. The breast milk produced in the first few days after birth. It has a slightly different composition to meet the needs of a newborn and is rich in antibodies, providing protection from infection.

contracture. Shortening of a muscle.

cord accident. An event that interrupts the flow of blood in the umbilical cord from the placenta to the baby. It could be the result of a knot in the umbilical cord, tearing of the umbilical cord, or compression of the umbilical cord.

corrected age. The age of a premature baby calculated from the due date (exactly 40 weeks). Corrected age accounts for the degree of prematurity.

corticosteroids. Also called steroids, are drugs that are similar to the hormone cortisol, which is produced by the adrenal gland. Corticosteroids reduce inflammation but also suppress the immune system. When given to a mother during pregnancy, corticosteroids improve lung maturity and have other positive effects for a premature baby.

cystic PVL. Cystic periventricular leukomalacia, or PVL, is a type of severe brain injury that is characterized by the loss of brain tissue around the ventricles. Cystic PVL occurs when so much tissue has been lost that cysts or holes develop in the brain.

delayed-interval delivery. Occurs in multiple pregnancies when labor stops after the first baby is delivered and there is a significant delay before delivery of the remaining baby or babies.

diastolic pressure. The lower number in a blood pressure measurement. It reflects the pressure in the blood vessels at the moment the heart is relaxed and filling with blood.

dichorionic/diamnionic twins. Twins who are in different amniotic sacs. Each baby is in a sac with two membranes (an amnion and a chorion). Dichorionic/diamnionic twins can be identical or fraternal.

directed donation. The process of giving blood in which the donor is giving blood for a specific person (referred to as recipient).

disseminated intravascular coagulation. A blood disorder that results in the inability of the blood to clot, potentially leading to uncontrolled bleeding.

domains. Components or aspects of social behavior.

donor twin. The smaller twin in twin-to-twin transfusion who donates blood to the recipient twin through a connection in the placenta.

durable medical equipment (DME). Medical equipment used at home, such as an oxygen saturation monitor, a feeding tube, or oxygen.

dystonia. Abnormal involuntary contractions of a muscle leading to twisting and tightness of muscle groups.

endotracheal tube. A tube inserted in the trachea (windpipe) to keep the airway open. It is connected to a ventilator to assist with breathing.

exchange transfusion. Removing blood that contains high levels of bilirubin and replacing it with donated blood that contains a normal level of bilirubin.

feeding residual. The amount of food left in the stomach before the next meal.

fetal fibronectin test. A test that identifies the presence of fetal fibronectin (which acts as a "glue" attaching the fetal sac to the uterus) in vaginal secretions. A positive test may indicate an increased risk of premature delivery in the next seven days. A negative test indicates the risk of premature delivery within the next seven days is less than 1 percent.

fontanelle. A soft spot in a baby's head between the bones of the skull. With time the skull bones grow and fuse together, closing the gap by 18 months.

full term. A pregnancy that delivers between 37 and 42 weeks.

fundoplication. Surgery in which the upper portion of the stomach (the fundus) is wrapped around the lower portion of the esophagus to treat severe gastroesophageal reflux (GER).

gastroesophageal reflux (GER). The backward flow of stomach acid and food from the stomach into the esophagus.

gastrostomy tube (G-tube). A feeding tube that is surgically implanted through the belly wall into the stomach.

germinal matrix. Specialized brain tissue that produces the nerve cells that become the cerebral cortex. The germinal matrix disappears between 34 and 35 weeks.

group B streptococcus (group B strep or GBS). A bacteria found in the vagina in approximately 25 percent of women during pregnancy. It is harmless to the pregnant mother but can cause serious infections for a baby, especially when premature.

hydrocephalus. Excess cerebrospinal fluid (CSF) in the brain. The pressure of the fluid can potentially damage the brain.

hydrops. Swelling in a baby before or after delivery.

hypertonicity. Increased muscle tone.

hypotonia. Decreased muscle tone.

hypoxic-ischemic encephalopathy. Damage to the brain caused by lack of oxygen and/or reduced blood flow to the brain.

indicated delivery. An induction or C-section for medical reasons.

inhaler. A handheld device that delivers a mist of medication to the lungs.

intubate. The placement of an endotracheal tube in the trachea (windpipe) to assist with breathing.

intrauterine growth restriction (IUGR). A condition in which a baby is smaller than expected (among the smallest 10 percent) during pregnancy.

isoimmunization. A condition during pregnancy in which the mother makes antibodies that cross the placenta and attack the baby's red blood cells.

kangaroo care. Holding a premature baby skin-to-skin.

left-to-right shunt. An abnormal flow of blood in the heart, causing oxygen-rich blood from the left side of the heart (destined for the brain and body) to be shunted back to the right side of the heart, where it mixes with oxygen-poor blood and heads back to the lungs again.

lower airways. Bronchi and bronchioles.

magnesium sulfate. A medication that may be given during pregnancy to stop preterm labor, prevent seizures in pre-eclampsia, and reduce the risk of cerebral palsy.

monochorionic/diamnionic twins. Identical twins with one outer membrane but two inner membranes.

monochorionic/monoamnionic twins. Identical twins in the same amniotic sac.

myelin. A fatty substance that coats the nerves, acting like insulation.

nasal cannula. Tubing used to deliver oxygen to the nose. One end attaches to an oxygen source and the other has two small prongs that fit in the nostrils.

nasogastric tube. A tube inserted through the nose to the stomach.

nebulizer. A machine that turns liquid medication into a mist for inhalation.

necrotizing enterocolitis. A condition in which, after a bowel is injured, bacteria leaks into the bowel wall.

neurologist. A doctor who specializes in disorders of the nervous system.

neuron. A nerve cell.

neurotransmitters. Chemicals that transmit and modify signals between neurons and between neurons and other cells.

neuroplasticity. The ability of the nervous system to change and adapt.

neurosurgeon. A surgeon who treats disorders of the nervous system.

NMDA receptor. A specialized receptor in the nervous system that plays a key role in the communication between neurons, especially in the brain.

opioid. A chemical that alleviates pain. Opioid medications, also called narcotics, are prescribed for pain control. The body also produces natural opioids.

orogastric tube. A tube inserted through the mouth to the stomach.

parasympathetic system. Part of the autonomic nervous system. Stimulation of the parasympathetic nervous system slows the heart rate and is important in digestion and elimination (urination and defecation). The actions of the parasympathetic system are sometimes described as "rest and digest."

peak flow meter. A handheld device that when blown into measures the ability to exhale. The measurement obtained is called the peak expiratory flow and is important in the management of asthma.

peripheral nutrition. Delivering nutrition via a smaller intravenous feed, typically in the hand or foot. Peripheral nutrition can meet some, but not all of the body's nutritional needs.

peristalsis. Involuntary contractions of the gastrointestinal tract that propel food through the esophagus, stomach, and bowel.

pertussis. Whooping cough, a highly contagious virus that infects the airways causing fits of coughing characterized by a "whoop" as air is inhaled.

phototherapy. Treatment of high bilirubin levels using specialized lights that convert bilirubin into a non-toxic substance.

PICC line (peripherally inserted central catheter). A long, central IV line inserted into a peripheral vein in the arm but ending in a larger vein in the chest, closer to the heart.

pneumothorax. A collapsed lung.

polyhydramnios. Excessive amniotic fluid.

preterm premature rupture of membranes (PPROM). Rupture of the membranes (breaking the water) before 37 weeks.

progesterone. A hormone produced during pregnancy. It can be used to treat cervical insufficiency. It can also be administered to prevent premature delivery in a woman who has a history of a premature delivery.

pulse oximeter. A machine that detects the concentration of oxygen in the blood.

recipient twin. The larger twin in twin-to-twin transfusion syndrome who constantly receives blood from the donor twin.

retinal detachment. A condition in which the retina partially or entirely peels away from the inside of the eye.

scleral buckle. Surgery to repair a retinal detachment. Material is sewn to the outside of the eye to apply pressure, keeping the retina flat against the inside of the eye.

seborrheic dermatitis. A condition that produces greasy, flakey scales on the scalp. In infants seborrheic dermatitis is also called cradle cap.

sensory integration disorder. A condition in which the nervous system does not process or interpret sensory input appropriately. As a result certain sensory experiences can be frightening, disturbing, or unpleasant.

surfactant. A fatty substance that coats the inside of the alveoli, preventing the air sacs from collapsing.

sympathetic nervous system. Part of the autonomic nervous system that mobilizes the body's defenses in response to stress. This is often called the "fight or flight" response. The sympathetic nervous system is always functioning, but activity increases with physical or emotional stress.

systolic pressure. The upper number in a blood pressure measurement. It is the maximum pressure in the arteries as the heart is contracting.

tardive dyskinesias. Involuntary and repetitive abnormal movements.

tocolytics. Medications to stop labor.

torticollis. Abnormal tightening of the neck muscles on one side of the body.

total serum bilirubin (TSB). The total amount of bilirubin in the blood.

trachea. Also called the windpipe: the tube that connects mouth and nose (upper airways) with the bronchi of the lungs.

transvaginal ultrasound. An ultrasound performed with a probe inserted into the vagina. This technique delivers clearer images of a baby in the first trimester of pregnancy and is the optimal method for evaluating the length of the cervix.

umbilical artery. An artery in the umbilical cord that transfers oxygen-poor blood from the baby to the placenta. There are usually two umbilical arteries.

umbilical vein. The vein in the umbilical cord that transfers oxygen-rich blood from the placenta to the baby.

unadjusted age. The age of a premature baby calculated from the date of birth. Also called chronological age.

upper GI series. An X-ray to evaluate the esophagus and stomach for physical abnormalities.

vitrectomy. Surgery in which some or all of the gel that fills the eyeball is removed. A vitriectomy may be performed in the case of retinal detachment.

ventricles. A system of fluid-filled cavities that connect within the brain. Cerebrospinal fluid (CSF) flows through the ventricles.

virus. A tiny infectious organism that can only replicate inside the cells of other organisms.

Index